P. 96 Ellis
P. 99
P. 82 Christ
P. 63 cognitive restructuring

# BEYOND CARL ROGERS

D1157960

# BEYOND
# CARL ROGERS

### EDITED BY
## David Brazier

CONSTABLE · LONDON

First published in Great Britain 1993
by Constable and Company Limited
3 The Lanchesters
162 Fulham Palace Road
London W6 9ER
Copyright © 1993 David Brazier and respective contributors
ISBN 0 09 472610 8
Set in Linotron Sabon 10pt by
Rowland Phototypesetting Limited
Bury St Edmunds, Suffolk
Printed in Great Britain by
St Edmundsbury Press Limited
Bury St Edmunds, Suffolk

A CIP Catalogue record for this book
is available from the British Library

# Contents

Part 3 · Towards the Future

# Introduction

## DAVID BRAZIER

Carl Rogers was a prophet of the personal approach to life. Now he is dead, but the need for the personal approach is no less pressing.

The forces of modernity have generally been those which seek to reduce persons to units. We live in mass societies in which bureaucracy can easily seem the most rational and just way of organizing life. Yet in this ever-expanding framework of rules and procedures, the person gets lost and the qualities which make persons different from machines are suppressed. The 'it' triumphs over the 'I and thou'.

Rogers had his roots in this modern world and began his work from a positivist, empirical foundation. He was thus able to speak the language of modern science and establish himself in the American academic world. The essential message which he gave out from this vantage point was, however, unremittingly one of respect for the power and importance of the personal.

It was within personal relationships that Rogers envisaged the way forward out of the disastrous dilemmas created by modernism. It was by enabling people from different cultural groups to appreciate each other's humanity that he believed the ending of war and genocide would come. It was by facilitating a real recognition of mutuality between individuals, from ordinary citizens to political leaders, that he believed genuine healing relationships could be established. It was by co-operating with those qualities like enthusiasm, emotional involvement and personal interest, which human beings do not share with machines, that he believed real education would prosper.

The bedrock of Rogers' philosophy was the notion that the

person is a living experiencing organism whose basic tendencies are trustworthy. It is still difficult for most people in the modern age to appreciate how revolutionary this simple idea is. It is not until we start to consider how much of our energy in modern society is spent on building and maintaining structures, the primary purpose of which is to eliminate the (dangerous) human element from human interactions, that we begin to get a glimpse of how radical Rogers' vision was and still is.

When people read about Rogers' ideas, it is not uncommon for them to think initially that there is nothing very remarkable about them. Do we not all believe in the importance of people being empathic to one another? What is so remarkable about that?

What is remarkable is that Rogers really meant it. And in carrying through what are essentially a very simple set of ideas whose rightness seems self-evident, he offers a challenge to the foundations of most of what modern life consists of.

The paradox is nowhere more apparent than when we look at the present state of counselling and psychotherapy itself. Rogers' ideas were revolutionary and intentionally so. The implications of his rejection of relationships based on power were immensely threatening to many established professional groups. Consequently, as the new profession of counsellor, which he did much to create, struggles to establish itself, it repeatedly runs into dilemmas and contradictions. Rogers believed that the therapeutic relationship was simply a special and intense form of the species of personal relationships in general. This, however, is not how the great majority of clients or professionals, including even those who purport to follow Rogers' philosophy, see it. Rogers believed in equalizing the power between providers and users of human services, but this principle of equality undermines the foundations upon which almost all such service institutions are founded. We cannot doubt that Rogers was serious in his principles. He stated them again and again throughout his life with unambiguous clarity. Those who feel inspired by him cannot escape the struggle of coming to terms with the implications.

When a leading thinker dies, those who have respected that

person's work experience a great mixture of reactions. The natural grief and sense of loss are likely to be translated into action of one kind or another. There is a new sense of responsibility for the work which has been begun. Now it is up to us. This is now the position for those who have been inspired by the work of Carl Rogers.

A number of reactions are possible. Some may feel that the important thing is to ensure that what Rogers established is not lost. People of this mind are likely to concern themselves with defining and preserving the pure form of what Rogers did and taught. These people perform a valuable service for us all in ensuring that something close to the way Rogers himself worked continues. There is, however, also a danger in this conservative stance. This danger is of the establishment of an orthodoxy within the person-centred approach, a result which would be the diametric opposite of what Rogers himself would have wanted. This is one of the prime paradoxes of Rogers' message. If we follow what he said, we are not following what he said, because what he said was that we should find our own way.

A similar but slightly different danger is that the radical potential of Rogers' inspiration will be smothered or simply go unnoticed and his ideas will be accommodated to pre-existing norms. Sigmund Freud, an earlier prophet of the personal dimension of life, was powerless to prevent his work being taken over by advocates of the medical model, which, in essence, was its complete antithesis. His work has been completely distorted in the process. Will Rogers fare any better? It is unfortunately the common fate of prophets of change to come to be regarded as eminent supporters of the establishment once they are dead. Will Rogers' influence come to be tamed in this way? On the other hand, it cannot be doubted that the influence of Freud has been revolutionary, even if not always in the ways he himself intended. This may well be the way it turns out with Rogers.

The question is, how to stay true to the essential message of the pre-eminent importance of the personal while carrying the work forward. How can we go beyond Rogers? One approach is that of cross-fertilization with other approaches. There are many theorists and practitioners today who are actively involved in the generation of integrated approaches to therapy. Some of the chapters in this volume do draw on another body of ideas, be it the arts, chaos theory, or comparative anthropology. Some may see this as a watering-down of the pure person-centred message but it can also be seen as the spreading of the basic principles into wider and wider fields.

Probably truer than either of these interpretations, however, is the intuition that we currently stand at a point of historical transition, a transition in our fundamental conceptualization of the world of our experience, and that Rogers was one, but only one, of the pivotal thinkers in this transition. Rogers believed that the actualizing tendency of the individual was simply a part of a greater actualizing tendency at work in society and indeed in the universe as a whole. It is not possible to disentangle whether individuals precipitate cultural change or whether the rise to prominence of the ideas of an individual is a function of a wider social need, but the sense that, as Rogers would say, 'something is happening' is palpable.

In the past few years there has thus been, and continues to be, a ferment of creative thought and experimentation among those who were most influenced by Rogers' work. For this creativity we must, in large measure, be grateful to Carl Rogers himself. He was never one to protect or restrict his approach. What seemed to please him most was when people came alive with their own contributions. It is important that his work and principles are not lost in the mêlée of developments which have come to fruit since his death, but it is also in keeping with his spirit that the tumult continue.

One purpose of this volume, therefore, is to put into more general circulation some of the most important contributions which have emerged from these debates recently. This book is not, however, simply an anthology. Although it contains a variety of viewpoints, it is not balanced nor representative. In keeping with the spirit of Rogers' work, it is a personal selection which aims to highlight the possibility that we may be moving into a more personal postmodern world, a world in which concern for one another will begin to take a higher priority than concern for control and order, and in which the uniqueness of each person will be valued more than the requirements of the system. The aim here, therefore, is that theory and humanity shall meet.

Rogers' conception of therapy was broad. He used the terms therapy, psychotherapy and counselling interchangeably, a usage which most of the contributors to this book follow. Beyond this, however, Rogers saw the therapeutic relationship as simply a special case of any form of good personal relationship and, like Freud, Jung and many other leading theorists before him, Rogers moved from the consideration of the therapy relationship itself to a consideration of the human situation in general.

This inevitably leads us to some fundamental questions about the nature of the person. Rogers entitled one of his most influential books *On Becoming a Person*, a tantalizing title which implies that a person is not simply something one is, but rather something which is the result of a process of becoming. The enigmatic nature of the self is the question to which Rogers' work repeatedly leads us. In this respect too, he seems to bridge two worlds. One pier of the bridge is firmly rooted, or so it at first seems, in traditional Western individualism. The goal of therapy is seen as individual independence and self-knowledge. But, as one delves further into his work, the notion of a self as real, fixed and knowable seems to slip away between the fingers. The 'fully functioning person' repeatedly described by Rogers seems actually to be one who is at ease with fluidity, a growing, changing, responsive being, full of possibilities, rather than a fixed character, and there is no ambiguity about the fact that Rogers believed this fully functioning person to be intrinsically social.

Rogers, then, was brought up in the 'modern' world but was able to open the door for us to a 'post-modern' universe. He provides a bridge between positivism and phenomenology. Rogers operated within a framework which people brought up to the assumptions of the scientific age could follow and appreciate, but which was shot through with post-positivist assumptions about the doubtfulness of definitive knowledge. Can we now establish a firmer footing in this new world? Or is that idea itself a contradiction of terms?

Not only was Rogers a bridge which arrived just at the time when many people felt a need to cross this particular river, but he was also an eminently crossable bridge. His writings were and are easily accessible, being repetitious, presented in short passages, in personal style. Although he managed to write cogently about a great range of subjects – counselling and psychotherapy, human relations groups, family relationships, education, organization theory, research, politics, community and peace studies – the main points that he made were always the same. What did Rogers write about? He wrote about empathy, congruence and positive regard. It was a simple message capable of a seemingly infinite variety of application. As a result, not only did many people cross this particular bridge, but all who did so acquired something memorable in the crossing, something which was both personal and universal, something which they could go on to apply in a great variety of different ways, each according to his or her situation.

For Rogers, it is the personal which is the key to the universal. To a modernist it seems absurd to think that large-scale problems can be solved by focusing upon single units. To those who have followed Rogers, however, it is clear that the human world is created by the perceptions, motives and intentions of persons and that if the person is devalued or discounted the outcome will be grim. If we accept the spirit of Rogers' work, we open ourselves to the possibility that the boundaries of the person are fluid, for we are all wrapped up in one another.

Just as Einstein introduced to physics the notion of relativity which cut away so many of the mechanistic assumptions upon which the subject had been previously established, so Rogers introduced to psychotherapy a phenomenological vision. He faced the implications of the realization that perceptions vary and no single reality can be isolated from the world's many observers and participants. Rogers helped us begin to approach this new more fluid universe, even though he was not always totally at home in it himself. Rogers opened a door to a view of psychology in which we no longer have to hold on to the idea of only one reality.

Post-Rogerian thinking is a product, in part, of the spread of Rogers' ideas outside the USA. Now we are increasingly aware of the differences of perspective to be found in the different cultures on this planet. It is no longer possible to doubt that different people see the world in different ways. And as soon as one allows this, it becomes apparent that even within one's own culture, every observer has his or her own standpoint from which more than just the perspective is different. Pluralism and diversity are now normal. The later part of Rogers' life was devoted to the cause of fostering understanding between members of different cultural groups. Now, an empathic appreciation of the standpoint of persons from other cultures is leading to a reassessment of the traditional Western conception of self upon which Rogers' work itself was originally founded.

Rogers' work was pre-eminently concerned with helping us to understand the 'frame of reference' of the other person, to understand the uniqueness of our own, and to appreciate rather than fear these differences. It was perhaps inevitable that work of this kind would lead to reconceptualizations of who we are and of how the world works. And the work is not finished yet.

In this volume, therefore, are gathered the writings of some of those who are currently involved in carrying forward the revolution which Rogers began. Nothing would have pleased him more than that we should be finding our own way beyond him. Although some of the contributions in this volume are implicitly at odds with some of the detail of his work, they are all very much inspired by its spirit. As editor, therefore, I very much hope that you, the reader, will be similarly inspired to go on beyond what is written here and to continue this creative process of generating a therapy for the century ahead and, beyond therapy, contributing to harmony between people generally, which Rogers saw as the necessary foundation for peace in the world.

# Part 1

## *The Core Conditions*

· 1 ·

# Authenticity, Congruence and Transparency

## GERMAIN LIETAER

Although Rogers had always attached great importance to the therapist's authenticity (see for example Rogers, 1951, p. 19), it was not until his 1957 paper about the 'necessary and sufficient conditions' that he mentioned it explicitly as a separate therapeutic condition, along with empathy and acceptance. From 1962 on, he even called it the most fundamental of all three basic attitudes, and continued doing this in his later works. Here is how Rogers describes it:

> Genuineness in therapy means that the therapist is his actual self during his encounter with his client. Without façade, he openly has the feelings and attitudes that are flowing in him at the moment. This involves self-awareness; that is, the therapist's feelings are available to him – to his awareness – and he is able to live them, to experience them in the relationship, and to communicate them if they persist. The therapist encounters his client directly, meeting him person to person. He is *being* himself, not denying himself.
>
> Since this concept is liable to misunderstanding, let me state that it does not mean that the therapist burdens his client with overt expression of all his feelings. Nor does it mean that the therapist discloses his total self to his client. It does mean, however, that the therapist denies to himself none of the feelings he is experiencing and that he is willing to experience transparently any *persistent* feelings that exist in the relationship and to let these be known to his client. It means avoiding the temptation

17

to present a façade or hide behind a mask of professionalism, or to assume a confessional-professional attitude.

It is not simple to achieve such reality. Being real involves the difficult task of being acquainted with the flow of experiencing going on within oneself, a flow marked especially by complexity and continuous change ... (1966, p. 185.)

This definition implies clearly that genuineness has two sides: an inner one and an outer one. The inner side refers to the degree to which the therapist has conscious access to, or is receptive to, *all* aspects of his own flow of experiencing. This side of the process will be called 'congruence'; the consistency to which it refers is the unity of total experience and awareness. The outer side, on the other hand, refers to the explicit communication by the therapist of his conscious perceptions, attitudes and feelings. This aspect is called 'transparency': becoming 'transparent' to the client through communication of personal impressions and experiences. Although this splitting up of genuineness into two components may be slightly artificial, we find it justified from a didactic point of view as well as clinically meaningful. Indeed, a congruent therapist may be very or minimally transparent, according to his style or orientation; a transparent therapist may be congruent, or he may be incongruent (something which makes him or her a 'dangerous' therapist). In a first point, we will discuss the concept of congruence, which has always been given the most weight in Rogers' definition. In a second one, we will then deal with transparency.

## 1. CONGRUENCE

Why did Rogers come to attach so much importance to the therapist's congruence, and why did he even come to see it as the most fundamental basic attitude? We hope to answer this question gradually, while further explaining the concept itself.

## PERSONAL PRESENCE

Rogers was always opposed to the idea of the therapist as a 'white screen'. He designed a 'face-to-face' type of therapy, in which the therapist is highly involved with the client's experiential world, and in which he, consequently, shows little of himself. Yet he does show his involvement in an open and direct way, without hiding his real feelings behind a professional façade. He tries to be himself without artificiality and haziness. By adopting such a 'natural', spontaneous attitude, the client-centred therapist certainly does not favour the process of regression and transference; but Rogers did not see this 'detour-process' as essential to personality change. More than the psychoanalysts, he believed in the therapeutic value of a 'real' relationship between client and therapist, and saw other, more important advantages in it as well. In such a working relationship, the therapist serves as a *model*: his congruence encourages the client to take risks himself in order to become himself. Along with this, Rogers gradually came to consider the therapist's congruence as a crucial factor in establishing *trust*, and came to emphasize the idea of acceptance and empathy only being effective when they are perceived as genuine:

Can I *be* in some way which will be perceived by the other person as trustworthy, as dependable or consistent in some deep sense? Both research and experience indicate that this is very important, and over the years I have found what I believe are deeper and better ways of answering this question. I used to feel that if I fulfilled all the outer conditions of trustworthiness – keeping appointments, respecting the confidential nature of the interviews, etc. – and if I acted consistently the same during the interviews, then this condition would be fulfilled. But experience drove home the fact that to act consistently acceptant, for example, if in fact I was feeling annoyed or skeptical or some other non-acceptant feeling, was certain in the long run to be perceived as inconsistent or untrustworthy. I have come to recognize that being trustworthy does not demand that I be rigidly consistent but that I be dependably real. The term 'congruent' is one I have used to describe the way I would like to be. By this I mean that whatever feeling or attitude I am experiencing would be matched by my awareness of that attitude. When this is true, then I am a unified or integrated person in that moment, and hence I can *be* whatever I deeply *am*. This is a reality which I find others experience as dependable. (Rogers, 1961, p. 50.)

This also means that the therapist should give priority to discussing his own feelings whenever they persistently stand in the way of the other two basic attitudes. Initially, Rogers considered such moments of self-expression as a 'help in need', as a therapist's last resort in discarding obstacles to his involvement with the client's experiential world. Gendlin, on the other hand, emphasizes more the gain, for therapist and client, resulting from daring to present oneself as 'not perfect':

'Congruence' for the therapist means that he need not always appear in a good light, always understanding, wise, or strong. I find that, on occasion, I can be quite visibly stupid, have done the wrong thing, made a fool of myself. I can let these sides of me be visible when they have occurred in the interaction. The therapist's being himself and expressing himself openly frees us of many encumbrances and artificialities, and makes it possible for the schizophrenic (or any client) to come in touch with another human being as directly as possible. (Gendlin, 1967a, pp. 121–22.)

The personal presence of the therapist should also be apparent from his concrete methodology, from the specific interventions and procedures used to facilitate and deepen the client's discourse. Important here is that the 'technique' should rest on an underlying attitude, that the therapist should stand behind it with his whole being (Kinget, 1959, p. 27), and that his work method should suit his personality. Rogers noticed 'with horror' in some of his pupils how reflecting feelings had deteriorated into aping, into a 'wooden technique', no longer carried by an inner attitude which emanates from an attempt to understand and check this understanding (Rogers, 1962, 1986; Bozarth, 1984). Rogers' view on the therapist's contribution thus increasingly evolved towards a *meta*theory, in which a number of basic attitudes are emphasized and in which concrete recipes and formulas of intervention have faded into the background. Gendlin writes about this evolution:

> Gone are formulas – even that most characteristic of client-centred modes of responding, which was called 'reflection of feeling'. As the term 'empathy' implies, we strive as always to understand and sense the client's feeling from his own inward frame of reference, but now we have a wider scope of different behaviors with which therapists respond to clients. In fact, I believe that it was in part the undesirable tendency toward formulas and stereotyped ways of responding which perhaps led Rogers to formulate this condition of 'congruence' as essential. (Gendlin, 1967a, p. 121.)

Because of the prime importance of the therapist's authenticity – but also perhaps because he was no great believer in the power of technique *per se* – Rogers thus emphasizes respect for each therapist's personal style. He does not want to put him in a methodological strait-jacket which would not suit his nature. That he is very broad-minded about this becomes obvious, for instance in his comment about the often widely diverging working methods of the therapists in the schizophrenic study:

> Perhaps the deepest of these learnings is a confirmation of, and an extension of, the concept that therapy has to do with the *relationship*, and has relatively little to do with techniques or with theory and ideology. In this respect I believe my views have become more, rather than less, extreme. I believe it is the *realness* of the therapist in the relationship which is the most important element. It is when the therapist is natural and spontaneous that he seems to be most effective. Probably this is a 'trained

21

humanness' as one of our therapists suggests, but in the moment it is the natural reaction of *this* person. Thus our sharply different therapists achieve good results in quite different ways. For one, an impatient, no-nonsense, let's put-the-cards-on-the-table approach is most effective, because in such an approach he is most openly being himself. For another it may be a much more gentle, and more obviously warm approach, because this is the way *this* therapist is. Our experience has deeply reinforced and extended my own view that the person who is able *openly* to be himself at that moment, as he is at the deepest levels he is able to be, is the effective therapist. Perhaps nothing else is of any importance. (Rogers, 1967a, pp. 185–86.)

As will be discussed further on, this respect for the therapist's own style is no passport to 'reckless experimenting'. Attention to the client's process and continuous following of his experiential track remain the ultimate guidelines for our interventions.

## CONGRUENCE AS *CONDITIO SINE QUA NON* OF ACCEPTANCE AND EMPATHY

After having examined the therapist's congruence from the angle of his 'personal presence', we now wish to inquire about the core meaning of the concept and discuss its importance for therapeutic work. Congruence requires, first of all, that the therapist be a psychologically well-developed and integrated individual, i.e. sufficiently 'whole' (or 'healed') and in touch with himself. This means amongst other things daring to acknowledge flaws and vulnerabilities, accepting the positive and negative parts of oneself with a certain leniency, being capable of openness without defensiveness to what lives in oneself and being able to get in touch with it, having a solid identity and a strong enough sense of competence, being able to function efficaciously in personal and intimate relationships without interference from one's own personal problems. Self-knowledge and ego-strength can perhaps be seen as the two cornerstones of this way of being (see e.g. McConnaughy, 1987).

Congruence is a correlative of acceptance: there can be no openness to the client's experience if there is no openness to one's own experience. And without openness there can be no empathy either. In this sense, congruence is the 'upper limit' of the capacity for empathy (Barrett-Lennard, 1962, p. 4). To put it differently: the therapist can never bring the client further than where he is himself as a person.

*Incongruence*

The importance of this attitude becomes especially clear when it is lacking, i.e. when the therapist is defensive and incongruent. Our personal difficulties may sometimes prevent us from letting the client's experience emerge fully, as it is. Life issues with which we have not dealt yet, personal needs which play along during therapy, personal vulnerabilities and blind spots, all may cause us to feel threatened and unable to follow with serenity certain experiences of our client (Tiedemann, 1975). To empathize with the experiential world of another person with values vastly different from our own, to let feelings of powerlessness and hopelessness emerge, to empathize with intense happiness, to deal without undue defensiveness with a client's intense negative or positive feelings towards us, all this is not easy. Because of our own experience of threat and defensiveness, there is a danger of us being so busy maintaining our own equilibrium that we break the deepening of the client's self-exploratory process either by keeping too much distance or by loosing ourselves in the other. Rogers puts it as follows:

> Can I be strong enough as a person to be separate from the other? Can I be a sturdy respecter of my own feelings, my own needs, as well as his? Can I own and, if need be, express my own feelings as something belonging to me and separate from his feelings? Am I strong enough in my own separateness that I will

not be downcast by his depression, frightened by his fear, nor engulfed by his dependency? Is my inner self hardy enough to realize that I am not destroyed by his anger, taken over by his need for dependence, nor enslaved by his love, but that I exist separate from him with feelings and rights of my own? When I can freely feel this strength of being a separate person, then I find that I can let myself go much more deeply in understanding and accepting him because I am not fearful of losing myself. (1961, p. 52.)

All this means that we, as therapists, need strong ego boundaries. An important part of being a therapist is to have the capacity to be steady as a rock (Cluckers, 1989): we sometimes have to pull the chestnuts out of the fire, deal with stormy emotions without being engulfed, deal constructively with hate and love without resorting to acting-out, deal with the client's praise and criticism of our own person; and we have to be able to tolerate ambivalence. To share empathically the other's world also implies putting our own world in parentheses, for the time being, and 'risking' personal change through contact with someone who is different from ourselves. Venturing in such an 'egoless state' (Vanaerschot, 1990) is easiest when we feel ourselves to be a sufficiently separate person with a well-defined personal structure and nucleus. Finally, we wish to point to a last aspect which demands a certain strength from the therapist: the fact that the client's discourse can be confronting to the therapist in so far as it addresses dormant issues in himself. Rombauts relates this being confronted with oneself to the kinship which exists between client and therapist, in the sense that both 'share a human existence'. He writes:

Because of this kinship, it is not only me who holds up a mirror to the client (although I find 'mirroring' a poor term), but also the client who holds up a mirror to me, showing me what I am, feel and experience. Dormant aspects of myself, which I have barely or not at all realized in my own life, can be touched upon and stirred up. As a consequence, I am constantly being confronted with myself when doing therapy, and led to question myself. Something happens, not only to the client but also to the therapist. We are companions-in-fate, in life as well as in therapy. (1984, p. 172.)

## Congruence and empathy

As we have seen, a lack of congruence undermines our therapeutic work. We can perhaps even better illustrate the importance of congruence from a positive angle or, at any rate, draw attention to a few aspects which we have not discussed yet, and which have a lot to do with the quality of our empathic interventions. A high level of congruence certainly guarantees a personal flavour to the communication of empathy so it would not be experienced by the client as a stilted application of technique. Indeed, the client finds himself faced with a therapist who is 'rooted' in his own experience, and who is, from there, trying to understand his message. The therapist not only summarizes the client's words, but puts into words 'what strikes him', what the client's discourse evokes in him, 'how it makes him feel', what he does not yet understand perhaps, but would like to understand, etc. Even though the therapist is in essence focused on the client's experiential world, the understanding is always a personal one, in the sense that his interventions originate in his own experience of what the client tells him. Occasionally (in my opinion very exceptionally) this can result in the therapist briefly mentioning an experience of his own, not in order to talk about himself or draw attention to himself, but as a way of letting the client know that he has been understood. This personalized form of empathy can perhaps best be illustrated by a couple of fragments from a session with 'A silent young man', where Rogers tries to share the feelings of hopelessness and rejection experienced by Jim Brown (see especially the T-interventions with an asterisk).

C: I just want to run away and die.
T: M-hm, m-hm, m-hm. It isn't even that you want to get away

from here *to* something. You just want to leave here and go away and die in a corner, hm?

(Silence of 30 seconds)

*T: I guess as I let that soak in I really do sense how, how deep that feeling sounds, that you – I guess the image that comes to my mind is sort of a, a wounded animal that wants to crawl away and die. It sounds as though that's kind of the way you feel that you just want to get away from here and, and vanish. Perish. Not exist.

(Silence of 1 minute)

 C: (almost inaudibly) All day yesterday and all morning I wished I were dead. I even prayed last night that I could die.

*T: I think I caught all of that, that – for a couple of days now you've just *wished* you could be dead and you've even prayed for that – I guess that – One way this strikes me is that to live is such an awful thing to you, you just wish you could die, and not live.

 . . .

 C: I ain't no good to nobody, or I ain't no good for nothin', so what's the use of living?

 T: M-hm. You feel, 'I'm not any good to another living person, so – why should I go on living?'

(Silence of 21 seconds)

*T: And I guess a part of that – here I'm kind of guessing and you can set me straight, I guess a part of that is that you felt, 'I tried to *be* good for something as far as he was concerned. I really tried. And now – if I'm no good to him, if he feels I'm no good, then that proves I'm just no good to anybody.' Is that, uh – anywhere near it?

 C: Oh, well, other people have told me that too.

 T: Yeah. M-hm. I see. So you feel if, if you go by what others – what several others have said, then, then you are *no good*. No good to anybody.

(Silence of 3 minutes, 40 seconds)

*T: I don't know whether this will help or not, but I would just

26

LIBRAIRIE
McGILL
BOOKSTORE

EC. # 001002000028     GST REG# R119128981           02/15/94
OMMIS/CASHIER 505

| SKU | QT. | Description | PRI. | TX | Extension |
|-----|-----|-------------|------|-----|-----------|
| 903754 | 1 | DEPRESSION AND | 4.95 | G | 4.95 |
| 820045 | 1 | ANXIETY AND ITS | 5.95 | G | 5.95 |
| 956465 | 1 | BEYOND CARL ROG | 19.99 | G | 19.99 |

|  |  |  |  | S/TTL | 30.89 |
|---|---|---|---|---|---|
| /TTL FOR GST | 30.89 | | | GST | 2.16 |
| /TTL FOR PST | 33.05 | S/T PST EXMP | 33.05 | | |
| PST S/TTL | 2.64 | – PST EXEMP: | 2.64 | PST | 0.00 |
| | | | | TTL | 33.05 |
| | | | | CA | 40.00 |
| | | | | CHANGE | 6.95 |

REMBOURSEMENTS: 10 JOURS AVEC CE RECU * REFUNDS: 10 DAYS WITH THIS RECEIPT

MERCI DE MAGASINER A MCGILL     01:45   THANK YOU FOR SHOPPING AT MCGILL

like to say that – I think I can understand pretty well – what it's like to feel that you're just *no damn good* to anybody, because there was a time when – I felt that way about *myself*. And I know it can be *really rough*. (Comment: This is a most unusual kind of response for me to make. I simply felt that I wanted to share my experience with him – to let him know he was not alone.)
(Rogers, 1967b, pp. 407–09.)

Deep empathy always means 'listening with the third ear', in which a regressive contact with one's own deeper feeling levels and the ability to imagine what one would feel in a similar situation are important elements. Rogers (1970) describes how he gradually developed more confidence in his own deeper intuitive levels:

I *trust* the feelings, words, impulses, fantasies, that emerge in me. In this way I am using more than my conscious self, drawing on some of the capacities of my whole organism. For example, 'I suddenly had the fantasy that you are a princess, and that you would love it if we were all your subjects.' Or, 'I sense that you are the judge as well as the accused, and that you are saying sternly to yourself, "You are *guilty* on every count."'

Or the intuition may be a bit more complex. While a responsible business executive is speaking, I may suddenly have the fantasy of the small boy he is carrying around within himself – the small boy that he was, shy, inadequate, fearful – a child he endeavors to deny, of whom he is ashamed. And I am wishing that he would love and cherish this youngster. So I may voice this fantasy – not as something true, but as a fantasy in me. Often this brings a surprising depth of reaction and profound insights. (p. 53.)

Gendlin too (1967b) describes how a therapist may empathically guess, on the basis of his own stream of thoughts and feelings, what the client is going through, or can try to evoke the felt sense of what the client says:

27

The patient talks, perhaps gets much value from having a friendly caring listener, but nothing of therapeutic relevance is said. There is only talk about hospital food, the events of the week, the behavior of others, a little anger or sadness, no exploration.

I become the one who expresses the feelings and felt meanings. I say, 'What a spot to be in' or, 'Gee, and they don't even *care* what *you* think about it,' or 'I guess that leaves you feeling help-less, does it?' or, 'Boy, that would make *me* mad,' or, 'It must be sad that he doesn't care more for you than *that*,' or, 'I don't know, of course, but I wonder, do you wish you *could* get mad, but maybe you don't dare?' or, 'I guess you could cry about that, if you let yourself cry.' (p. 398.)

All this goes to show that congruence and empathy are not oppo-sites. On the contrary, empathy is always implicitly carried by the therapist's congruence: we always understand the other via our-selves, through our kinship as fellow human beings (see Vanaer-schot, 1990). So far we have discussed the importance of congruence mainly in the context of acceptance and empathy for the client's experiential world, disregarding the interaction here-and-now. However, empathy for what happens *between* client and therapist, for the kind of relationship pattern which they create in their influence on each other, is an equally important aspect of the process, and here too – maybe especially here – the therapist's congruence is crucial. Indeed, here it functions as an 'interactional barometer' for what happens in the relationship. We will discuss this aspect later, under the heading 'Transparency'.

IMPLICATIONS FOR TRAINING AND PROFESSIONAL PRACTICE

Personal maturity, together with the basic clinical aptitudes related to it, can thus be considered as the therapist's main instrument in client-centred therapy. In this respect, we share the view of psycho-analysts. It should thus not come as a surprise that, in our training, special attention is paid to the personal development of the thera-

pists-to-be. We are, of course, not talking here about 'direct training' in congruence, but about the slower and indirect ways of
personal therapy and personalized supervision, in which the person
of the therapist is as much focused on as the client's process. As
far as personal 'didactic' therapy goes, I myself am strongly in
favour of participation in intensive long-term group therapy.
Indeed, therapeutic experience in a group offers, more than individual therapy, the possibility of observing one's own interpersonal
functioning, something which is crucial for therapeutic work (see
also Bolten, 1990). Individual therapy may then remain highly
desirable, along with group therapy, but it may not be essential for
every trainee.

The willingness to work on one's own personality development
should not be limited to the training period, but should be viewed
as a 'life task'. Therefore, regular peer-review, either within one's
own team or outside it, seems highly desirable. A sufficiently safe
atmosphere is however a must, in order to allow the taking of
personal risks and the acceptance of a vulnerable position. In a
broader sense, we, as therapists, should take special care of ourselves, and watch out for signs of overburdening, loneliness, alienation, and of getting stuck in personal problems. When our need is
too big, we may not have enough energy left to turn towards our
client with serenity. What could we then do to avoid such impasses?
'Caring' for one's own personal relationships, re-entering therapy
before it is too late, cutting one's workload and making time to be
with oneself . . . may, besides supervision, already achieve a great
deal. Exceptionally, changing an appointment with a client may be
indicated. Besides this, it may help a great deal to 'prepare' oneself
before an interview. Rombauts writes about this:

> It seems important that I stop all my other activities, even if only
> a few minutes before, in immediate preparation for the contact
> with a client. I try as much as possible to step out of my own
> world, and let my worries and concerns fade into the back-
> ground. I also concentrate mentally on my client, for example
> by recalling our last session, but also more generally by letting

him be present, as it were, with everything he evokes in me in terms of memories and feelings. To use Gendlin's terms, I turn towards the 'felt sense' for the client, which lives in me.

In this way, I try to increase my receptivity towards the client, and remove as much as possible any lack of openness I may feel. However, should I not have succeeded, the first few moments of the session are often enough to create more openness, not only towards my client but also towards myself. There exists thus an interaction: the state of fundamental openness in my personal world is the soil on which the contact with the client grows; but also, this contact, this therapeutic involvement, highly enhances the quality of the openness in my personal world. (1984, p. 170.)

All this leaves us perhaps with the impression that the therapist should be a 'superman'. But this is not what Rogers and others had in mind. It is indeed so that someone who wants to become a therapist has to be prepared to go through life paying sufficient attention to his own inner life and his way of relating to others. He also has to be, generally speaking, quite sturdy. This however does not mean that he could not have problems which may at times be quite acute. The important point here is not to avoid these problems, to dare scrutinize them, to remain open to critical feedback, to learn to see how one's difficulties interfere with one's therapeutic work, and to do what is needed to remedy the situation. It is furthermore important to get to know and accept with leniency our own limits: we do not have to be able to work well with *all* types of clients. We may try to change our limits, but learning to know and accept them is not an unimportant task during training and beyond.

And, to conclude, I want to mention this: client-centred literature contains little in the way of the concrete forms which incongruence can take. As a process-oriented theory of therapy, it emphasizes mainly the formal signals. We can see this, for example, in Barrett-Lennard's definition of incongruence:

Direct evidence of lack of congruence includes, for example, inconsistency between what the individual says, and what he implies by expression, gestures, or tone of voice. Indications of discomfort, tension, or anxiety are considered to be less direct but equally important evidence of lack of congruence. They imply that the individual is not, at the time, freely open to awareness of some aspects of his experience, that he is lacking in integration and is, in some degree, incongruent. (1962, p. 4.)

In the psychoanalytic literature, however, a great deal is said about the diversity in content of 'countertransference reactions' and their psychogenic roots; the interested reader may find a great deal in the following publications: Glover, 1955; Groen, 1978; Menninger, 1958; Racker, 1957; Winnicott, 1949.

## 2. TRANSPARENCY

### ITS PLACE IN THE EVOLUTION OF CLIENT-CENTRED THERAPY

At the beginning of this paper, I have described transparency as the outer layer of authenticity: the explicit communication by the therapist of his own experiences. It should however be mentioned that, even without the use of such explicit 'self-revelations', the client-centred therapist is fairly transparent to his client, and that the distinction we made between congruence and transparency should not be understood in absolute terms. Our client gets to know us through everything we do and don't do, be it verbal or non-verbal. Especially in client-centred therapy, where the working relationship is heavily coloured by personal involvement with the client on the basis of one's own experience of the moment, the client is likely to get to know who the therapist is, as a person. We can thus never function as a white screen. Each therapist evokes slightly different feelings in his clients, and this is perhaps an important element in the success or failure of a therapy, an element which surpasses concrete methods and interventions: does the client meet a therapist whose personality and way of being-in-the-world allow him to move, precisely at the level where his own problem lies? We have but little control over this aspect of therapy, and research on the topic of treatment recommendations yields but little useful information on this topic.

As to the therapist's self-expressive interventions in the narrow sense of the word, it is remarkable how reluctantly they were introduced and accepted in the evolution of client-centred therapy. This should not surprise us. Indeed, it belongs to the nuclear identity of client-centred therapy that the therapist follow his client *within the client's own frame of reference*. However, between 1955 and 1962 this principle became more flexible. Client-centred therapy evolved from 'non-directive' to 'experiential', and this allowed the therapist to bring in something from his own frame of reference, as long as he kept returning to the client's experiential track (Gendlin, 1970). This was thus the context in which self-expressive interventions became accepted. Thus, we deal here with interventions where the therapist starts from his own frame of reference, as is also the case in interpretations, confrontations and proposals for the use of particular techniques, for instance. Gradually, the expression of personal feelings became no longer restricted to being a 'help in need', i.e. used in cases where the therapist could no longer genuinely accept and empathize, but it became thought of as having *positive potential* for deepening the therapeutic process. What the therapist experiences in contact with his client is now considered as important material and potentially useful for the client in his exploration of himself and his relationship patterns (for a thorough analysis of Rogers' evolution in this regard, see Van Balen, 1990). And Rogers attributes, in a more general way, a modelling function to the transparency of the therapist as well.

It is not easy for a client, or for any human being, to entrust his most deeply shrouded feelings to another person. It is even more difficult for a disturbed person to share his deepest and most troubling feelings with a therapist. The genuineness of the therapist is one of the elements in the relationship that make the risk

32

of sharing easier and less fraught with dangers. (1966, pp. 185–86.)

Three factors seem to have played a role in this evolution. First of all, there was the study with schizophrenics which Rogers and his colleagues carried out between 1958 and 1964. With this very withdrawn group of patients, the 'classical' type of intervention – reflection of feelings – fell short: there was often very little to reflect. In their attempts at establishing contact, the client-centred therapists learned to use an alternative source of help, their own here-and-now feelings:

> When the client offers no self-expression, the therapist's momentary experiencing is not empty. At every moment there occur a great many feelings and events in the therapist. Most of these concern the client and the present moment. The therapist need not wait passively till the client expresses something intimate or therapeutically relevant. Instead, he can draw on his own momentary experiencing and find there an ever-present reservoir from which he can draw, and with which he can initiate, deepen, and carry on therapeutic interaction even with an unmotivated, silent, or externalized person. (Gendlin, 1967a, p. 121.)

There was, moreover, the contact with a number of existential therapists, such as Rollo May and Carl Whitaker, who criticized them for effacing themselves too much in the therapeutic relationship, for standing too much behind the client as an *alter ego* and too little as a real other person with an own personal identity. Thus Whitaker gave the following comments on a number of excerpts from client-centred therapies with schizophrenics:

> It is as though the two were existing in some kind of common microcosm or isolation chamber or like twins in utero. These interviews are intensely personal for both of these individuals but only the patient's life is under discussion. This is so distinct that one sometimes feels there is only one self present and that

self is the patient. It is as though the therapist makes himself artificially miniature. Sometimes this is so dramatic that I almost feel he disappears. This is in specific contrast to our type of therapy in which both persons are present in a rather specific sense and the therapeutic process involves the overt interaction of the two individuals and the use of the experience of each of them for the patient's growth. (Rogers *et al.*, 1967b, p. 517.)

This 'willingness to be known' (Barrett-Lennard, 1962, p. 5), which had gradually found its way into their individual therapy praxis, emerged even more forcefully (perhaps at times too forcefully) in the 'encounter movement' of the sixties and seventies (Rogers, 1970, pp. 52–55). Group dynamics, with its emphasis on 'feedback in the here-and-now', was certainly not foreign to this. All these influences have made client-centred therapy into a more inter-actional one, with the therapist not only functioning as an *alter ego*, but also as an independent pole of interaction, who expresses, at times, to the client his own feeling about the situation. On account of this transparency, the process becomes more a dialogue, an I-Thou encounter. (Buber and Rogers, 1957; Van Balen, 1990, pp. 35–38.)

In such an authentic mutual encounter, there may be moments in which the therapist almost relinquishes his professional role and encounters the client in a very personal and profoundly human way. According to Yalom, such 'critical incidents' often become turning-points in therapy. He believes that they are seldom mentioned in the psychiatric literature out of shame, or out of fear of censorship; they are also seldom discussed with trainees because they do not fit the 'doctrine' or because one is afraid of exaggerations. Here are a couple of Yalom's many examples (1980, pp. 402–03):

A therapist met with a patient who during the course of therapy developed signs suggesting cancer. While she was awaiting the results of medical laboratory tests (which subsequently proved negative) he held her in his arms like a child while she sobbed and in her terror experienced a brief psychotic state.

For several sessions a patient had been abusing a therapist by attacking him personally and by questioning his professional skills. Finally the therapist exploded: 'I began pounding the desk with my fist and shouted, Dammit – look, why don't you just quit the verbal diarrhea and let's get down to the business of trying to understand yourself, and stop beating on me? Whatever faults I have, and I do have a lot of them, have nothing to do with your problems. I'm a human being too, and today has been a bad day.'

## TRANSFERENCE AND TRANSPARENCY

Working through of the transference is not thought of as a nuclear process, as the 'pure gold', in client-centred therapy. The therapeutic relationship is not structured in such a way as to maximize regression. We rather follow an orthopedagogic model, in which growth is stimulated right from the start, and the *real* relationship aspects are emphasized. John Shlien even goes as far as to say that transference is 'a fiction, invented and maintained by therapists, in order to protect themselves from the consequences of their own behaviour' (Shlien, 1987, p. 15). But, with the reviewers of his paper and with such authors as Pfeiffer (1987) and Van Balen (1984), we have to say – in my opinion – 'Yes, John, there is a transference.' Or as Gendlin has it:

If the client is a troubled person, he cannot possibly fail to rouse difficulties in another person who relates closely with him. He cannot possibly have his troubles all by himself while interacting closely with the therapist. Necessarily, the therapist will experience his own version of the difficulties, twists, and hang-ups which the interaction must have. And only if these do occur can the interaction move beyond them and be therapeutic for the client. (Gendlin, 1968, p. 222.)

35

In client-centred therapy too, the client repeats his past in his relationship with the therapist. But the way it is dealt with is partly different from the psychoanalytic orientation. Firstly, there is the belief that certain transference reactions – which can be viewed as security measures on the part of the client – will gradually melt away without explicit working through under the beneficial effect of a good working alliance. Secondly, client-centred therapy does not provide a *priority in principle* to working with a problem in the here-and-now relationship with the therapist. The criterion for further exploration is, according to Rice, the vividness with which a certain type of problem is experienced, and not where this experience is located on the triangle here-elsewhere-in the past:

> In a real sense, any member of a class is as worthwhile exploring as any other. Neither the past nor the present has priority, but rather the vividness with which an experience can be recounted by the client. After all, the more vividly an experience is re-counted, the more likely it is to be an experience that is emotion-ally important to the client. More adequate processing of any one experience should lead to more adaptive responses in a whole range of specific situations. (1974, p. 303.)

In Rice's view, therefore, the working through of transference reac-tions in the here-and-now of the therapeutic relationship is not a 'must' but a possibility, a sub-process along with other ones. I personally feel that it is nevertheless an important sub-process which comes into prominence especially in the longer therapies. What is then the role of the therapist's transparency when transfer-ence reactions are worked through in client-centred therapy? Here are some thoughts.

The emphasis is not on working to achieve insight, which consists of recognizing and genetically understanding how the client distorts the therapist and relates to him in a structure-bound way, but on the corrective emotional experience:

It isn't enough that the patient *repeats* with the therapist his maladjusted feelings and ways of setting up interpersonal situations. After all, the patient is said to repeat these with everyone in his life, and not only with the therapist. Thus, the sheer repeating, even when it is a concrete reliving, doesn't yet resolve anything. Somehow, with the therapist, the patient doesn't *only* repeat; he gets *beyond* the repeating. He doesn't only *re*live; he lives *further*, if he resolves problems experientially. (Gendlin, 1968, p. 222.)

This 'living further' sometimes requires more than neutral benevolence (Wachtel, 1987). It requires the therapist not to present himself as a white screen but – apart from, and in addition to, his empathic interventions – to deal in a transparent way, at the right moment, with what lives in the interaction between the two of them, and hereby to express *his* version of the interaction. Thus, the therapist may question the client's image of him by putting his own experience next to it. He may give the client feedback about his way of dealing with him and about the feelings he evokes in him. Where needed, he makes his own limits explicitly known: indeed the client can 'discuss' anything; he cannot just do anything. In order to perform this interactional work properly, a therapist should pay special attention to what happens *between* him and his client, to the relationship aspect of the communication; and he should keep in touch with what the client 'does to him'. In Yalom's words, the here-and-now feelings are to the experienced therapist 'of as much use as a microscope is to the microbiologist' (1975, p. 149). We also find this view in the humanistic branch of the Freudian analytic school, where the 'countertransference' is not seen as a 'crack in the mirror', but as an aid in the analytic work (Corveleyn, 1989; Wachtel, 1987). Obviously we could find here a link with the interactional approach, as proposed by Kiesler (1982) as well as by van Kessel and van der Linden (1991).

SUGGESTIONS FOR PRACTICE

What can a therapist reveal and what not? And at what moment can this best be done? Rogers dismisses this question – perhaps wisely – with the very general answer, '. . . when appropriate' (1962, p. 417). Wachtel too, a psychoanalyst, writes in the same vein: 'I wish there were hard and fast rules about when exactly such self-revelations are helpful. Unfortunately, there are none . . .' (1987, p. 183). We are thus thrown back on our general clinical feeling and our common sense. This does not mean, however, that there are no guidelines. Indeed, there is the basic criterion which always goes back to the following question: does our self-revelation serve the client's growth process (Yalom, 1980, p. 414)? Can our client use and integrate this information? In other words, we are talking here about a transparency with responsibility, and this includes right away the presence of important restrictions. As therapists, we have to withhold what does not help the client, and this is a lot. Yalom illustrates this basic principle with a touching story about two famous healers, taken from a book by Hermann Hesse.

> Joseph, one of the healers, severely afflicted with feelings of worthlessness and self-doubt, sets off on a long journey to seek help from his rival, Dion. At an oasis Joseph describes his plight to a stranger, who turns out to be Dion; whereupon Joseph accepts Dion's invitation to go home with him in the role of patient and servant. In time Joseph regains his former serenity, zest, and effectance and becomes the friend and colleague of his master. Only after many years have passed and Dion lies on his deathbed does he reveal to Joseph that when the latter encountered him at the oasis, he, Dion, had reached a similar impasse in his life and was *en route* to request Joseph's assistance. (Yalom 1975, p. 215.)

From this focus on the client's growth process it follows that the therapist will only exceptionally mention facts from his personal life. But 'exceptionally' does not mean 'never'. A therapist can thus, as said earlier, reveal something about himself as a way of showing empathy. Also, when a personal event in his life comes to weigh heavily on his therapeutic work (such as the death of an important person), it may be better to mention it. And what if the client asks us for our personal philosophy of life, our lifestyle or our values? Obviously, we should be very careful here and explore, with the client, the precise meaning of his question. In most cases the client is not really interested in the therapist, but such questions may be situated within the search for a solution to a personal problem, or within a specific relational context. Our attention should thus go in that direction. Client-centred therapists generally refrain from giving 'personal testimony', in my opinion for good reason: indeed, the client has to find his *own* way. But one thing does not always exclude another. We should not forget that clients often obtain indirect clues as to 'how we live our lives' and that we can never totally escape a modelling role. This is not wrong in itself, at least not if we can bring the client to becoming independent from it. If we succeed in this, the client gradually comes to see his therapist as 'a fellow pilgrim' (Yalom, 1980, p. 407), with whom and against whom he can clarify his own choices. This happens mostly towards the end of therapy, i.e. in the existential phase (Swildens, 1988, p. 54), in which the client has reached the point where he can choose freely.

As will be clear from what I said before, self-revelation has seldom anything to do with the therapist's personal past or present life. But what can the therapist then reveal? The answer is obvious: his feelings towards the client in the here-and-now, towards what happens in the session between both of them. Here too, the therapist remains sober. Only 'persisting' feelings count, and besides, the therapist has to ask himself if the moment is appropriate. There is thus a problem of 'timing': is there a chance for the client to be sufficiently receptive to my feedback about how I experience the interaction, or should other therapeutic tasks take precedence? Sometimes the relationship has not yet acquired enough security and solidity, and this should be worked on first. In moments of great vulnerability, empathic closeness is perhaps all that is needed.

Sometimes, the client may first need a chance to fully express his feelings towards the symbolic figure of the therapist, without immediately being 'stopped' by a confrontation with the 'reality' of how the therapist experiences it himself . . . But occasionally, the therapist's experience of the interaction may be the most fruitful approach to deepening the process.

Besides the question of what can be said and when, we also should address the one about *how* to communicate our own experiences in the most constructive way. Here are some suggestions from the client-centred literature: Boukydis, 1979; Carkhuff and Berenson, 1977; Depestele, 1989, pp. 63–69; Gendlin, 1967b; Gendlin, 1968, pp. 220–25; Kiesler, 1982; Rogers, 1970, pp. 53–57. All illustrate how important it is that the therapist's self-expressive interventions be supported by the basic attitudes. The close bond with congruence is obvious: the feeling for what happens in the relationship, the interactional barometer, thus should function properly! This presupposes a close contact with one's own flow of experiencing and the meanings which it may contain, sufficient awareness of what may be one's personal contribution to the difficulties arising in the relationship, and when needed, sufficient openness to facing the issue in question (so it would not become a battle about who is right), being capable of communicating one's experience in a process-compatible way, i.e. in all its complexity and changingness. As an example of the latter, Rogers describes how a therapist can communicate 'boredom':

But my feeling exists in the context of a complex and changing flow, which also needs to be communicated. I would like to share with him my distress at feeling bored and my discomfort in expressing it. As I do, I find that my boredom arises from my sense of remoteness from him and that I would like to be in closer touch with him; and even as I try to express these feelings they change. I am certainly not bored as I await with eagerness, and perhaps a bit of apprehension, for his response. I also feel a new sensitivity to him now that I have shared this feeling which has been a barrier between us. I am far more able to hear the surprise, or perhaps the hurt, in his voice as he now finds himself speaking more genuinely because I have dared to be real with him. (1966, p. 185.)

Along with this, there is the link with unconditional positive regard. Self-expressive confrontations are most effective when embedded in, and communicated out of, deep involvement with the person of the client. Consequently, it is important for the therapist not to let negative feelings accumulate for too long, so as to remain sufficiently open to the client. He further has to let it be known clearly that his feelings have to do with a specific behaviour of the client's, and not with the client as a person. Therefore, the therapist's feedback should be as explicit and concrete as possible: how the feeling took shape and what precisely in the client's way of interacting has brought it on. Perhaps most importantly, the therapist should remain focused on the positive life-tendencies behind the client's disturbing behaviour and behind his own negative feelings, and communicate these as well. Thus, in our earlier example, Rogers communicates the inside, the reason for his boredom, which is his desire for more contact with the client. When we give a client feedback about a behaviour which irritates us, we try to get in touch with the needs and positive intentions behind it, and include these in our discussion. Gendlin gives the following example of this, pertaining to setting limits:

For example, I might not let a patient touch me or grab me. I will stop the patient, but in the same words and gesture I will try to respond positively to the positive desire for closeness or physical relations. I will make personal touch with my hand as I hold the patient away from me, contact the patient's eyes, and declare that I think the physical reaching out is positive and I welcome it, even though I cannot allow it. (I know at such times that I may be partly creating this positive aspect. Perhaps this reaching is more hostile, right now, than warm. But there is warmth and health in anyone's sexual or physical need, and I can recognize that as such.) (1967b, p. 397.)

Finally, we should always take care in maintaining the process sufficiently client-centred and making it a 'self-revelation without imposition'. This can best be done by letting the influencing occur as openly as possible. Two 'rules of communication' should be remembered here. The first one, to use Rogers' words, is 'owning' or giving I-messages instead of you-messages: the therapist indicates clearly that he is the source of the experience and tries above all to communicate what he himself feels, rather than making evaluative statements about the client. He will, for example, not say 'How intrusive of you' but 'When you called me for the second time this week, I felt put under pressure and as if taken possession of . . .' The second rule of communication is, in Gendlin's words, 'always checking' or 'openness to what comes next': after each intervention – and especially after one which originated in our own frame of reference – tuning in anew to the client's experiential track and continuing from there. All these suggestions should make it clear that constructive self-revelation is far removed from acting-out. It is rather a form of 'disciplined spontaneity' which, along and together with empathy, constitutes a second line from which the client can evolve towards a 'further living' inside and outside of therapy, towards new and more satisfactory ways of dealing with himself and others. Mistakes may, of course, occur if self-revelation is used rather carelessly, but to leave out this important reservoir of relationship information could be equally detrimental: an omission which could lead to substantial reduction in quality of the therapeutic process.

REFERENCES

BARRETT-LENNARD, G. T. (1962), 'Dimensions of therapist response as causal factors in therapeutic change', *Psychological Monographs*, 76 (43, Whole No. 562).

BOLTEN, M. P. (1990), 'Opleidingstherapie en de plaats van groepen', *Tijdschrift voor Psychotherapie*, 16, 60–68.

BOUKYDIS, K. N. (1979), 'Caring and confronting', *Voices. The Art and Science of Psychotherapy, 15*, 31–34.

BOZARTH, J. D. (1984), 'Beyond reflection: Emergent modes of empathy', in R. F. Levant and J. M. Shlien (eds.), *Client-Centered Therapy and the Person-Centered Approach: new directions in theory, research and practice* (pp. 59–75). New York: Praeger.

BUBER, M., and ROGERS, C. R. (1957), 'Dialogue between Martin Buber and Carl Rogers', in H. Kirschenbaum and V. L. Anderson (1989), *Carl Rogers: Dialogues* (pp. 41–63). Boston: Houghton Mifflin.

CARKHUFF, R. R., and BERENSON, B. G. (1977), 'In search of an honest experience: confrontation in counseling and life', in R. R. Carkhuff and B. G. Berenson, *Beyond Counseling and Therapy* (pp. 198–213). New York: Holt, Rinehart and Winston.

CLUCKERS, G. (1989), ' "Containment" in de therapeutische relatie: de therapeut als drager en zingever', in H. Vertommen, G. Cluckers, and G. Lietaer (eds.), *De Relatie in Therapie* (pp. 49–64). Leuven: Leuven University Press.

CORVELEYN, J. (1989), 'Over tegenoverdracht gesproken: hinderpaal of hulpmiddel?', in H. Vertommen, G. Cluckers, and G. Lietaer (eds.), *De Relatie in Therapie* (pp. 103–19). Leuven: Universitaire Pers Leuven.

DEPESTELE, F. (1989), 'Experiëntiële psychotherapie: een stap in de praktijk', *Tijdschrift Klinische Psychologie, 19*, 1–15 en 60–81.

GENDLIN, E. T. (1967a), 'Subverbal communication and therapist expressivity: Trends in client-centered therapy with schizophrenics', in C. R. Rogers and B. Stevens, *Person to Person* (pp. 119–28). Lafayette, Ca: Real People Press.

GENDLIN, E. T. (1967b). 'Therapeutic procedures in dealing with schizophrenics', in C. Rogers *et al.* (eds.), *The Therapeutic Relationship and its Impact: a study of psychotherapy with schizophrenics* (pp. 369–400). Madison: University of Wisconsin Press.

GENDLIN, E. T. (1968), 'The experiential response', in E. F. Hammer (ed.), *Use of Interpretation in Therapy: technique and art* (pp. 208–27). New York: Grune and Stratton.

GENDLIN, E. T. (1970), 'A short summary and some long predictions', in J. T. Hart and T. M. Tomlinson (eds.), *New Directions in Client-Centered Therapy* (pp. 544–62). Boston: Houghton Mifflin.

GLOVER, E. (1955), *The Technique of Psycho-Analysis*. New York: International Universities Press.

GROEN, J. (1978), 'Spiegels en schaduwen van de analyticus', *Tijdschrift voor Psychotherapie*, 1, 19–27.

KIESLER, D. J. (1982), 'Confronting the client-therapist relationship in psychotherapy', in J. C. Anchin and D. J. Kiesler, *Handbook of Interpersonal Psychotherapy* (pp. 274–95). New York: Pergamon.

KINGET, M. (1959), 'Deel I. Algemene presentatie', in C. R. Rogers and M. Kinget, *Psychotherapie en Menselijke Verhoudingen* (pp. 11–171). Utrecht/Antwerpen: Spectrum and Standard.

LIETAER, G., ROMBAUTS, J., and VAN BALEN, R. (eds.), *Client-Centered and Experiential Psychotherapy in the Nineties*. Leuven: Leuven University Press.

MCCONNAUGHY, E. A. (1987), 'The person of the therapist in psychotherapeutic practice', *Psychotherapy*, 24, 303–14.

MENNINGER, K. A. (1958), 'Transference and countertransference', in K. A. Menninger, *Theory of Psychoanalytic Technique* (pp. 77–98). New York: Basic Books.

PFEIFFER, W. M. (1987), 'Uebertragung und Realbeziehung in der Sicht klientenzentrierter Psychotherapie', *Zeitschrift für Personenzentrierte Psychologie und Psychotherapie*, 6, 347–352.

RACKER, H. (1957), 'The meanings and uses of countertransference', *Psychoanalytic Quarterly*, 26, 303–57.

RICE, L. N. (1974), 'The evocative function of the therapist', in D. A. Wexler, and L. N. Rice (eds.), *Innovations in Client-Centered Therapy* (pp. 289–311). New York: Wiley.

ROGERS, C. R. (1951), *Client-Centered Therapy*. Boston: Houghton Mifflin.

ROGERS, C. R. (1957), 'The necessary and sufficient conditions of therapeutic personality change', *Journal of Consulting Psychology*, 21, 97–103.

ROGERS, C. R. (1961), *On Becoming a Person*. Boston: Houghton Mifflin.

ROGERS, C. R. (1962), 'The interpersonal relationship: the core of guidance', *Harvard Educational Review*, 32, 416–29.

ROGERS, C. R. (1966), 'Client-centered therapy', in S. Arieti (ed.), *American Handbook of Psychiatry* (Vol. 3, pp. 183–200). New York: Basic Books.

ROGERS, C. R. (1967a), 'Some learnings from a study of psychotherapy with schizophrenics', in C. R. Rogers and B. Stevens, *Person to Person* (pp. 181–91). Lafayette, Ca: Real People Press.

ROGERS, C. R. (1967b), 'A silent young man', in C. R. Rogers *et al.* (eds.), (1967a), op. cit. (pp. 401–16).

ROGERS, C. R. (1970), *On Encounter Groups*. New York: Harper and Row.

ROGERS, C. R. (1986), 'Carl Rogers's column: reflection of feelings', *Person-Centered Review*, 1, 375–77.

ROGERS, C. R. *et al.* (eds.), (1967a), *The Therapeutic Relationship and its Impact: a study of psychotherapy with schizophrenics*. Madison: University of Wisconsin Press.

ROGERS, C. R. *et. al.* (1967b), 'A dialogue between therapists', in C. R. Rogers *et al.* (eds.), (1967a), op. cit. (pp. 507–20).

ROMBAUTS, J. (1984), 'Empathie: actieve ontvankelijkheid', in G. Lietaer, Ph. van Praag, and J. C. A. G. Swildens (eds.), *Client-Centered Psychotherapie in Beweging* (pp. 167–76). Leuven: Acco.

SHLIEN, J. (1987), 'A countertheory of transference', *Person-Centered Review*, 2, 15–49 (comments: 153–202/455–75).

SWILDENS, H. (1988), *Procesgerichte Gesprekstherapie*, Inleiding tot een gedifferentieerde toepassing van de cliëntgerichte beginselen bij de behandeling van psychische stoornissen. Leuven, Amersfoort: Acco/De Horstink.

TIEDEMANN, J. (1975), 'Angst in de therapeutische relatie', *Tijdschrift voor Psychotherapie*, 1, 167–71.

VANAERSCHOT, G. (1990), 'The process of empathy: holding and letting go', in G. Lietaer, J. Rombauts, and R. Van Balen (eds.), op. cit. (pp. 269–93).

VAN BALEN, R. (1984), 'Overdracht in client-centered therapie. Een eerste literatuurverkenning', in G. Lietaer, Ph. H. van Praag, and J. C. A. G. Swildens (eds.), *Client-Centered Psychotherapie in Beweging* (pp. 207–26). Leuven: Acco.

VAN BALEN, R. (1990), 'The therapeutic relationship according to Carl Rogers: only a climate? A dialogue? Or both?', in G. Lietaer, J. Rombauts, and R. Van Balen (eds.), op. cit. (pp. 65–86).

VAN KESSEL, W., and VAN DER LINDEN, P. (1991), 'De-hier-en-nu relatie met de therapeut: de interaktionele benadering', in J. C. A. G. Swildens, O. de Haas, G. Lietaer, and R. Van Balen (eds.), *Leerboek Gesprekstherapie: de cliëntgerichte benadering*. Amersfoort/Leuven: Acco.

WACHTEL, P. L. (1979), 'Contingent and non-contingent therapist response', *Psychotherapy: Theory, Research and Practice*, 16, 30–35.

WACHTEL, P. L. (1987), 'You can't go far in neutral: on the limits of therapeutic neutrality', in P. L. Wachtel, *Action and Insight* (pp. 176–84). New York: Guilford.

WINNICOTT, D. W. (1949), 'Hate in the countertransference', *International Journey of Psychoanalysis*, 30, 69–74.

YALOM, I. D. (1980), *Existential Psychotherapy*. New York: Basic Books.

YALOM, I. D. (1975), *Theory and Practice of Group Psychotherapy* (rev. ed.). New York: Basic Books.

# · 2 ·

# Empathy as Releasing Several Micro-Processes in the Client

## GREET VANAERSCHOT

### INTRODUCTION

Within psychotherapy, Rogers considered empathy to be crucial as one of the three core conditions which the therapist's relationship offer must meet, so that the client can use this relationship for constructive personality change (Rogers, 1957). Since Rogers' first formal definition in 1957, the concept has gone through many changes and elaborations as a result of developments within the client-centred theory and therapy, instigated by, among others, Gendlin and Rice. The view of empathy as presented here tries to integrate these several visions. I will describe empathy from three points of view: those of the therapist, the observer and the client. These three points of view are analogous to the three phases of the empathy cycle described by Barrett-Lennard (1981).

From the therapist's point of view, empathy is described as a specific inner listening attitude, a special way of being that is characterized by a 'process-like' way of functioning. The observer's point of view refers to the communication of empathy. I will be quite short on these two points of view, not at all because there is not much to say about them, but, since space is limited, I think it makes more sense to deal with one point of view elaborately, namely that of the client.

## EMPATHY AS AN ATTITUDE

When describing empathy as an attitude, we will deal with the inner process that takes place in the empathically listening therapist. From the therapist's viewpoint, empathy is a special way of knowing. The therapist tries to get to know the client's inner world. But one can never directly know someone else's inner world. 'Knowing' in this context means, that the therapist's inner phenomenological world and state of mind, which he can indeed directly perceive, are as similar as possible, or more, are almost identical to the client's. The therapist achieves this by gradually tuning in to the client. This 'tuning in' takes place by comparing signals, coming from (relayed by) the client, with referents in himself. These signals from the client may be non-verbal utterances as well as the articulation of the client's feelings. Examples of inner referents include both the therapist's own experiences and feelings which are similar to the client's, and knowledge of other phenomenological worlds acquired through films, literature, therapy experience, learning about psychopathology, and so on. On the basis of his own inner referents, the therapist will come to, or set up, hypotheses about the client's inner world. In this process of tuning in the therapist uses his imagination, his phantasy, as if he were to place himself in the client's shoes. 'Putting oneself in the place of', '*zich verplaatsen in*' are characteristic descriptions of this imaginative process that is so typical in any understanding of another person's state of mind. When Rogers uses the expression 'as if', I think that we can understand this as referring to the vicarious or substitutive aspect, which is an essential element in the empathic process.

In the empathic experience therapist and client together jointly experience what the client is expressing. The therapist will come to this 'experiencing-together' by using his own inner referents that are evoked by the client.

A simple example: A client is weeping. What the therapist directly observes are tears, dropping from the client's eyes, the client's breath sticking in his throat, moaning. The therapist compares these signals with his own referents, in this case with his own experience that weeping is an expression of pain and sorrow. The therapist thus comes to a hypothesis about the client's affective state. He is experiencing, together with his client, some of the client's pain and sorrow. This, however, does not mean a unification or merging with the client. Empathy is not emotional identification: the therapist himself as a person does not experience these feelings for he is only experiencing this pain and sorrow temporarily, that is, restricted to the contact with the client, and the therapist is continuously aware of the fact that those feelings belong to the client and are not originating from himself. This keeping distance, not merging with is also indicated by Rogers' 'as if' condition.

But the feelings and state of mind that the therapist evokes on behalf of the client's signals are but hypotheses, which must be checked with the client's phenomenological world. The therapist does so by expressing his empathic understanding. From the therapist's viewpoint, communicating the inner understanding means checking the hypotheses which he has formed about the client's world: the empathic response is a way of testing. It is a necessary step in the tuning-in process, through which the therapist comes to an as exact and intensive sharing as possible. In this way, the therapist is checking whether or not, he sees and feels accurately. That is, he is checking his own experiencing with the client's. And then, the client's reaction to the therapist's reflection enables the therapist to correct his understanding, to tune in better and more sensitively to his client. The important aspect of the therapist's attitude is not the fact that, in his contact to the client, the therapist eliminates himself as a person, but the very way in which he applies himself.

The therapist uses his own person in such a way that he is fully open, completely receptive to what is coming from the client. This openness is no passive 'state', the therapist is not an empty box that lets itself be filled with the other. This openness is, as Rombauts (1984) puts it, an active receptiveness.

The activity that is meant here refers to a double move. On the one hand, the therapist is looking for referents in himself which seem similar to what he is perceiving (sees, hears, feels) with the client. On the other hand, he has to loosen those referents from the particular structure and context they have for himself. This double move is necessary in order to understand the client. If the therapist does not make the first move, namely looking for referents in himself, then he can hear what the client is saying, but it does not get through to him, he does not understand the meaning of it. If the therapist is indeed appealing to his inner referents, but neglects to separate them from the particular context and structure which they have for himself, then there is a real danger that the therapist is merely understanding himself and following his own track instead of understanding the client in his individuality and uniqueness. The therapist usually makes those moves without thinking about it, almost automatically. Only when difficulties occur in this respect, does it become clear that the therapist has neglected to make one of these moves. An example can help to clarify this process: the case of a client who has extreme difficulties in expressing what is going on in herself. She is often blocked, because she is clearly overwhelmed by intense emotions. At a particular moment in the session, she says, 'Like a steamer, that's how I feel.' The therapist responds, 'A steamer . . . that evokes in me the feeling of as if there were an enormous pressure inside, as if something is about to explode. Is that what you are feeling?'

What has now been going on in the therapist? The therapist has looked for referents inside herself that helped her to understand what the client might feel inside. It is of course only an assumption, because she cannot be sure about it until she notices the client's response, in this case: a visibly relieved agreement. Important here is that the therapist has not applied these referents with the structure and context they have for herself. For the image of a steamer is, in the therapist's experience, linked to a series of pleasant memories. Aside from the contact with the client, the word 'steamer' evokes a warm feeling in the therapist. It reminds her of the summer holidays during which she helped her grandmother sterilizing and preserving vegetables. The threatening aspect of the steamer is, in her experience, but a marginal comment rather emphasizing the safe feeling of 'being with grandmother' than attacking it. And yet it is this very connotation of threat and danger that the therapist is appealing

RELEASING SEVERAL MICRO-PROCESSES IN THE CLIENT

to, but then undone of the particular context and structure it has for the therapist herself. And that's exactly why we consider this response as empathic.

It is the disconnecting of the referents from one's own specific context and structure that makes any understanding an empathic understanding. The inner attitude which is the basis of empathic understanding, consists in the therapist using himself in a fluid and flexible way. This means that he is using referents in himself, loose from his own personal experience and meaning structure. In other words, the therapist needs to have 'pure, unadulterated' referents at his disposal. No meanings are drawn on, which are not there for the client. Or, if this is indeed the case, those meanings need to be open to correction by the client. An example in which this is not the case can help to clarify this.

As a child, a therapist had a very problematic relationship with her mother, in the sense that her mother was a very warm and understanding person, but at the same time very controlling and possessive. This results in our therapist always experiencing intimacy and warmth tied up with control and power, and what is more she always takes care to keep enough distance in her own intimate relationships. Well, this therapist starts seeing a client who did miss that 'warm nest' experience and who is continuously looking for a 'good mother' to compensate this lack. The therapist feels threatened by the relational demand of the client, and she will do anything to divert the client from her 'sickly' demand for intimacy.

Due to our therapist not being able to disconnect, in her experience, warmth and intimacy from power and control, although she may know very well in theory that these feelings need not go together, our therapist cannot follow the client accurately. She cannot counsel the client truly in her search for intimacy, and will neglect all utterances of the client that could correct her understanding. In fact, this therapist does not respect her client in her uniqueness, but is responding merely out of her own problem.

## THE EMPATHIC RESPONSE

When describing the different forms of expressing empathic understanding, one is supposed to take the position of an observer of the therapeutic event. In other words, when listening to a tape or video-recording of a therapeutic session, which interventions can then be called empathic? Or course, the empathic response can never be seen apart from the breeding ground from which it originated, namely the therapist's inner process. Nor can the empathic response be considered loose from the impact it has on the client. This, however, does not mean that one could not try to describe the explicit verbal response. Several authors have described different ways of responding, which can be considered empathic.

Thus there is the 'reflection of feeling', well known as the typical client-centred response. On the other hand, there is the experiential response, as described by Gendlin (1968), and the evocative reflection and the empathic prizing, both described by Rice (1974, 1990). The experiential response, as well as the evocative reflection and empathic prizing, are further elaborations of the reflection of feeling. Client-centred therapists felt the urge to look for and formulate further differentiations of the reflection of feeling, in order to identify the active aspect in this type of response, because the three core conditions described by Rogers as necessary and sufficient for personality change were, within the psychotherapeutic world, indeed accepted as necessary, but not as sufficient. As a consequence, client-centred therapy was in imminent danger of being absorbed by other schools that thought the client-centred method suitable to create a climate of confidence, useful only as the background for other interventions. There was a danger that practitioners might lose sight of the fact that client-centred therapy is powerful and active in itself.

Some of Rogers' staff members and students started emphasizing the process theory (Gendlin, 1968, 1970, 1974; Rice, 1974, 1983, 1984). They tried to identify and analyse the ways through which clients could come to a change. They did so in order to describe clearly the therapeutic interventions which facilitate those changes.

They had often had many years of experience with the reflection of feeling, which was their starting point, and they sought to identify those ways of reflection, those therapeutic interventions that make a client indeed work effectively.

The therapist, however, can also look for other, more idiosyncratic ways to communicate his empathic understanding. Some of these are described by Bozarth, in his article 'Beyond reflection, emergent modes of empathy' (1984).


## RECEIVED EMPATHY, OR EMPATHY BASED ON THE EXPERIENCE OF THE PERSON EMPATHIZED WITH

Now let me turn to my main topic, which is empathy from the client's viewpoint. 'How does it feel to be empathized with?' is the question. In this respect we may recall that Barrett-Lennard discusses three phases in the empathic circle, the third being: 'received empathy, or empathy based on the experience of the person empathized with' (Barrett-Lennard, 1981, p. 95). Barrett-Lennard refers here to the important condition established by Rogers that the client must be able to perceive the therapist's empathy. This condition seems obvious, but it is often overlooked.

Rogers (1957) wrote:

> The final condition as stated is that the client perceives, to a minimal degree, the acceptance and empathy which the therapist experiences for him. Unless some communication of these attitudes has been achieved, then such attitudes do not exist in the relationship as far as the client is concerned, and the therapeutic process could not, by our hypothesis, be initiated. Since attitudes cannot be directly perceived, it might be somewhat more accurate to state that therapist behaviours and words are perceived by the client as meaning that to some degree the therapist accepts and understands him. (p. 99.)

The question that arises then is: if the client perceives the therapist's empathy, what impact does this have? In other words: what is the therapeutic effect of empathy? Is empathy a primary relationship factor or a task-relevant factor (Rice, 1983)? Is the therapeutic effect of empathy due to a climate it creates or to the direct effect of the concrete empathic response?

It must be clear now that we cannot speak of one single therapeutic consequence of empathy, but that several micro-processes are induced in the client, and it is these I wish to describe.

## CONSEQUENCES OF AN EMPATHIC CLIMATE

The therapeutic effect of empathy as a primary relationship factor always implies the presence of the other core conditions. Unconditional positive regard and congruence are part of the empathic involvement and of the empathic response of the therapist (Wexler, 1974; Rogers, 1975). The empathic response is the most important way for the therapist to communicate acceptance, dedication, warmth and real commitment to the client. What, then, is the experiential impact of such a real and accepting empathic climate?

### 1. ONE FEELS VALUED AND ACCEPTED AS A PERSON

The therapist can only be really empathically involved in the client's world when he values him as the person that he is, namely as a seeking human being with his very own capacities to develop and grow. This means that the therapist is – in a certain way – really concerned about his client and that he really cares for him. One cannot be a good therapist unless one really cares about people; unless one can be touched when one's client makes some progress; unless one can feel happy with the little steps that the client takes; unless one can give support to the client's growth process.

The client experiencing all this in relation to his therapist gradually starts to experience himself as worthwhile. He learns to value himself as a person, not only because he is doing well at work or because he always does what others ask him to do, but because he also learns to care for himself. Barrett-Lennard puts it as follows:

> Being listened to and heard, particularly in the context of struggle and felt limitation, helps to validate and empower us. We see ourselves in the other's mirror and know our humanity and that we are not alone. We see that our image is many-sided and changing and feel a movement toward new possibilities. Implicit is an element of healing or growth. (1988, p. 419.)

## 2. ONE FEELS CONFIRMED IN ONE'S EXISTENCE AS AN AUTONOMOUS, VALUABLE PERSON WITH ONE'S OWN IDENTITY

The empathizing therapist confirms the client in his right to exist. Acquiring the feeling: 'I may exist' is at stake here, and this is a more fundamental and more existential experiential learning than the feeling of being worthwhile which has been mentioned before. Every human being feels the urge to have his existence confirmed by others. Recognition by another is the basis to develop one's own identity. In this respect, Rogers quotes Laing, saying that 'the sense of identity requires the existence of another by whom one is known'. (Rogers, 1975, p. 139.)

## 3. ONE LEARNS TO ACCEPT ONE'S OWN FEELINGS

Empathy is non-judgemental. The empathic therapist does not condemn, does not judge. The client experiences that he is allowed to feel and express anything, without destructive consequences, without the therapist rejecting him. Thus self-acceptance is facilitated. To put it with Rogers (1975): 'If I am not being judged, perhaps I am not so evil or abnormal as I have thought. Perhaps I don't have to judge myself so harshly.'

## 4. EMPATHY DISSOLVES ALIENATION

When the client feels that what he is talking about apparently makes sense to the therapist, there is a double result. The client's experience not only becomes more meaningful to himself, it also gives him the feeling that he is not so abnormal, so different and so strange as he had, originally, feared.

Rogers describes this experience as follows:

> I have been talking about hidden things, partly veiled even from myself, feelings that are strange – possibly abnormal – feelings I have never communicated to another, nor even clearly to myself. And yet, another person has understood, understood my feelings even more clearly than I do. If someone else knows what I am talking about, what I mean, then to this degree I am not so strange, or alien, or set apart. I make sense to another human being. So I am in touch with, even in relationship with, others. I am no longer an isolate. (Rogers, 1975, p. 7.)

Rogers suggests that this might explain one of the major findings of the schizophrenic research project in which those patients who were counselled by an explicit empathic therapist showed the sharpest reduction in schizophrenic pathology.

## 5. ONE LEARNS TO TRUST ONE'S OWN EXPERIENCE

The empathizing therapist concentrates on and is guided by the client's experiential track. The client thus learns to focus on his own experiencing, and he experiences through the course of therapy that he can rely on it and that his acting can be guided by it.

This is a capacity, which will also be useful later on, in handling new problems. Client-centred therapy does not work on the symptoms, but also teaches the client to deal with himself and the world in another, experiential way. Thus:

Many people who come for therapy see themselves as venturing into life without an adequate guidebook, either rigidly following certain routes on the basis of external criteria or approaching each new choice feeling that they lack the necessary data for making a decision. Yet for many decisions the crucial data lie in the inner awareness of what it would really feel like in either direction. If clients can get in touch with this inner awareness and begin to use it as a trustworthy guide, they can more confidently take control of their own lives. (Rice, 1983, p. 44.)

## THE IMPACT OF THE CONCRETE EMPATHIC RESPONSE

Having considered empathy as setting a climate, let us now turn to its task relevance. Rice (1983) defines the task-relevant relationship factors as those which enable the client to engage productively in different approaches to exploration and growth. In any therapy the client engages in a series of therapeutic tasks which we can consider as constituent components of the entire therapeutic process. The task-relevant relationship factors are those aspects of the relationship interactions that facilitate or even induce those therapeutic tasks. Meant here is the therapeutic relationship as a working relationship. The therapist's empathy is not merely an important primary relationship factor, but it also substantially facilitates certain tasks, certain micro-processes and it is these micro-processes we will elaborate on now.

There are two main groups: 1. the deepening and facilitating of experiencing, and 2. cognitive restructuring. Of course there is a theoretical distinction for didactic purposes. In the complex reality of therapy, these two are closely linked, and it is rather a matter of emphasis.

## 1. DEEPENING AND FACILITATING THE EXPERIENCING

Rogers wrote that:

> When persons are perceptively understood, they find themselves
> coming in closer touch with a wider range of their experiencing.
> This gives them an expanded referent to which they can turn
> for guidance in understanding themselves and in directing their
> behaviour. If the empathy has been accurate and deep, they may
> also be able to unblock a flow of experiencing and permit it to
> run its uninhibited course. (Rogers, 1975, p. 8.)

In Rogers' description of this experiencing-deepening and experi-
encing-facilitating process that is started off by feeling oneself
empathically understood, we can distinguish two micro-processes
as follows:

### i) *Getting in more direct and close touch with*

An important impact of the empathic response is that it helps the
client to get more in touch with what he is saying and feeling at
that particular moment. We consider this to be one of the major
functions of accurate empathy of the first level. Accurate reflections
of feeling help the client to get more in touch with the meaning of
what he is trying to say; with the full emotional load that his words
imply. 'You are to bring to life what is only being talked about',
is Martin's advice to the therapist (Martin, 1983). The accurate
reflection of feeling is slowing down the client's narrative. As such,
the client gets, so to say, the time and the opportunity for his own
words to affect him, to resonate within himself and as such to
experience their impact fully.

In this way the therapist is also helping his client to face really
what he has just said. In this sense, the empathic response is at the
same time confronting too. Martin (1983) compares the work of
the empathic therapist to a painter making a picture. The therapist

gathers all (is taking) the material the client has brought up in bits and pieces, putting it all together as a vivid picture and holding it in front of the client, asking, 'Look, this is what you've said. We have to look at it in all its complexity and confusingness. Look.' (Martin, 1983, p. 32.) Furthermore, accurate reflections of feeling do help the client to feel more sharply and clearly what he actually wants to express. After an accurate paraphrase, or even after a word by word restatement of what the client has said, the therapist often gets the reaction: 'That's not what I mean, it's more like . . .' Let's hope that the therapist then does not react with 'But you have just said it yourself!', but that he will be wise enough to understand that what was true a minute ago, doesn't fit any longer with the client's experiencing right now.

Experiential responding means that the therapist's response is aimed at the source where the words are coming from, and not at the words themselves. This is exactly the process the client is going through. The client too is getting more in touch with the source his words are coming from; that's why he can articulate more accurately what could be expressed only vaguely before. Gendlin (1970) calls this an important phase in the process of focusing, namely, the direct referent on the bodily felt meaning that is a direct entrance way to the experiencing.

> If he is understandingly listened to and responded to, he may be able to refer directly to the felt meaning which the matter has for him. He may then lay aside, for a moment, all his better judgement or bad feeling about the fact that he is as he is, and he may refer directly to the felt meaning of what he is talking about. He may then say something like: 'Well, I know it makes no sense, but in some way it does.' Or: 'It's awfully vague to me what this is with me, but I feel it pretty definitely.' (Gendlin, 1970, p. 142.)

In this quotation, an important constituent process of this getting more in touch with the inner experiencing comes up, namely: the therapist's empathic involvement, expressed through the empathic response, protects the client's inner reaction against a sort of inner critic who wants to put aside the felt sense as senseless, unrealistic, self-destructive or ridiculous. This enables the client to refer directly to his inner experiencing. He can for instance say, 'It feels as if something terrible and terrifying is going to happen to me. But this is of course ridiculous. You just have to accept such things. But nevertheless, that's how it feels, a sort of panic.'

When the client, counselled by an empathically responding therapist, manages to keep his attention directly upon his conceptually vague, but nevertheless definitely perceptible inner reaction, he might be able to conceptualize some main aspects of it. Once the client has conceptualized some main aspects of his felt sense, he does usually experience more strongly and vividly the felt meaning of it. He also gets more enthusiastic and hopeful about this process of direct referring to himself. The direct referring to his own inner felt sense is more and more appreciated as: 'I am in touch with myself.'

Getting more in touch with oneself is a confronting, but at the same time a very relieving process. It is confronting because often the client has to deal with issues that evoke feelings of discomfort, vague anxiety or not-feeling-well; uninviting topics for discussion, so to speak.

But nevertheless, the paradox is that, once the client has decided to bring up an unpleasant topic, and comes to focus his attention on the felt sense of what he is talking about, his anxiety seems to ease. The more the client comes to conceptualize correctly some aspects of this frightening feeling, the more the anxiety gives way to relief. Directly referring to the felt meaning leads to a bodily felt relief in itself.

Summarizing all this, one may state that the client, through listening to the therapist 'repeating' his utterances, gets the opportunity (space and time) to let his own words resonate. So he can get more in touch with the source his words are coming from, and, out of this contact with his own bodily felt experiencing, he can articulate more sharply and definitely what he wants to express (cf. 'getting more sharply in touch with' in Rice and Greenberg, 1990).

## ii)  Coming to new aspects of one's experiencing

The empathic response brings the client into contact with aspects of his experiencing he was hardly aware of before, as it helps the client to get through himself further and further into the jungle of his experiencing. Especially the deep empathic response can induce this micro-process. By 'deep empathic response', I am referring to advanced empathy, empathic guessing, empathic non-understanding, explorative questions, try-sentences, experiential response, evocative reflection. The empathic response helps to explicate the implicit. Sometimes, the empathic response can actively complete the experiencing, namely when the client himself meets with a wall in exploring his own experiencing and is off the track completely. Thus, the empathizing therapist contributes in an active way to the unblocking of the client's experiencing. He can offer a correct symbolization that can bring certain aspects of the implicit experiencing in process again: the right word or the right question at the right time.

In therapy, the client focuses on his experiencing, more particularly on his felt sense: an unclear, concrete, bodily feeling that pushes for explication. The felt sense is, so to speak, the contact point, at a given moment, with the implicitly functioning experiencing. The felt sense the client is touching at that very moment comes into interaction with symbols (a word, an image, something the client reaches himself or that is offered by the therapist). Implicit meanings are explicated. The complement also happens. A symbol can bring a part of the implicitly functioning experiencing into process in the form of a concrete felt sense, that again can unfold in new symbols. And it is this process we are discussing here.

For instance: A client came into therapy with complaints about 'feeling bad' in the sense of feeling ill. She complained about dizziness, stomach aches, qualms and other physical symptoms that she herself experienced as anxiety. So in therapy she started exploring what this overwhelming anxiety was about, where it came from, what it meant, and so on. At a particular moment in therapy when the client once again was telling her therapist how extremely bad she had felt that week, the therapist drew the client's attention to the fact that 'feeling bad' can also mean: feeling wrong. So the therapist gives another meaning to the client's statement, namely 'bad' in the context of morals, of good or bad. This evokes a lot in the client. A series of memories, about feeling sinful and bad when doing something her parents or the schoolteacher did not like, came back to her.

So feeling bad seemed to be the physical translation, so to speak, of the client's self-image. And that self-image, those implicit meanings, became available for the client, or to put it otherwise: were brought into process by the therapist's input. And since the client himself is often not capable of offering this fitting symbolization to himself, the therapist's contribution in this respect must undeniably be called process-stimulating. For the interaction between feeling and symbols, that would stagnate without the therapist's input, can now go on. So the client gets more access to his experiencing, comes in touch with a more extended part of his experiential world, and becomes in that sense more congruent too.

Gendlin (1970) calls this process 'unfolding'. The experiencing unfolds by a gradual step-by-step explicating of the felt sense, as well as by a sudden 'opening up', whereby the client experiences a great physical relief and a sudden knowing. Often this knowing is preconceptual: the client has not yet found the words to tell what it is he 'has got', but he knows that he can indeed say.

The unfolding of the felt sense does not bring a solution; explicating the implicit does not solve the problems. But nevertheless, something has changed. What was felt before, seems to have more sense now. For instance: the vaguely felt anxiety that was evoked by a particular situation, and for which there seemed to be no reason, has now become pretty understandable. 'Of course, that's why I am so afraid,' the client realizes.

Once the problem is tabled in that way, something can be done about it too. And even if there is not an immediate solution, even then something has changed, namely the relief of being understandable to oneself, of being more in touch with oneself. Out of this newly acquired self-knowledge, the same situations and problems can be experienced or handled differently. The same situation can be more easily accepted, for instance.

Explicating implicit experiential aspects or meanings 'at the edge' of 'conscious' experiencing, can be very confronting. For instance: A client is telling his therapist how he withdraws when having a rough time, then lets his feelings rage out in himself. Here he uses the image of a safe place in which he retires. The therapist invites the client to describe that place. The client chooses the image of a dungeon in a medieval fortress: thick, solid walls, quiet, no sound, no intruders, safe. The therapist reflects on this, but also mentions something of what the image of the dungeon evokes in himself, namely: cold, dark and particularly desolate and lonely. The client reacts very touched and shocked, as if his breath were cut off. Here he comes in touch with his enormous loneliness which he had tried to deny to himself for so many years. The therapist's empathic reflection brings the client into contact with an experience that is indeed very painful, and which helps him to experience more sharply his vague feelings of discontentment, and to see more clearly what they are about.

## 2. COGNITIVE RESTRUCTURING

The empathic response has also an important function in the cognitive information processing the client is living through. For the empathic response contributes to the client processing better the information that is coming to him from both inside and outside sources. Wexler, the most important exponent of the cognitive trend, considers the therapist to be a 'surrogate information processor' (Wexler, 1974, p. 97). The therapist performs this function by means of his empathic responding. An empathic response, Wexler said, is an attempt to organize and articulate the meaning of the information the client is processing. A good empathic response offers the client a structure that more fully captures, and better organizes, the meaning of the information that the client is processing, than the structure the client had generated himself.

An example may help to clarify this (Martin, 1983, p. 36). A client says, 'A lot of the time it seems like people are . . . I don't know . . . really mean . . . no, not mean . . . they're loving, I guess . . . at least some . . . like some I know.' The therapist might respond, 'I'm not sure I got all that, but let me try. It sounds confusing . . . trying to know how you feel about the way people are toward you. The ones that matter to you seem to be loving, you guess, but at the same time that doesn't seem quite the whole truth because they seem mean in some ways too. Is that close to what you mean?' The therapist is structuring the client's incoherent speech, and in doing so, he is also structuring the client's experience.

What then in a good empathic response makes for the facilitating of the information processing? To put this question differently: What are the properties, then, of a good empathic response that lead to a better processing of the client's experience?

Here we can discern three micro-processes, three different ways through which empathic responding can facilitate better information processing. These are (i) focusing the client's attention, (ii) recall, and (iii) organizing information. When the client's utterances suggest the presence of an automated and constricted pattern of schematic processing, then the therapist will react with an empathic response that can induce one of these three micro-processes.

Concrete examples of process-markers that indicate such automated and constricted processing are: describing a complex experience in a packaged or condensed fashion; connotative expressions that are rich in subjective meanings, not easily understandable to the therapist; and stereotypic qualifiers of the 'ought' and 'should' variety (Toukmanian, 1990, p. 313).

## i) Focusing the client's attention

Empathic interventions aimed at those process markers that suggest constricted information processing focus the client's attention on such expressions using paraphrases, reflections or bids for clarification (Toukmanian, 1990, p. 313; Wexler, 1974). The empathic response focuses the client's attention on certain information facets the client is not attending to himself. The client tends to select those facets of meaning that can most readily be organized within his existing rules and schemes. This results in the client leaving relevant information out for subsequent processing, and it will often be precisely that kind of information that might change the client's interpretation and experience of the given situation.

An example: Someone who experiences men as authoritarian, punishing and aggressive will be inclined to see in every man only those aspects, and will neglect the co-operative and tender sides.

Another example: A client is always talking about the responsibilities womanhood brings, the heaviness of it and the anxiety that is evoked in her by the thought of taking on all those responsibilities. But she never mentions the positive side of it, namely that she can take her own decisions, may choose for herself, have more freedom to do what she wants herself, whenever she wants to do it, and in the way she wants to. When the therapist confronts her with all this, she at first reacts in a very surprised way. But the more this idea really 'sinks in', the more relief she experiences.

Given the limited capacity of short-term memory, it frequently happens that the client slightly touches some information, but loses sight of it due to the presence of other information impinging on him. So it is the therapist's task to refocus the client's attention on what would otherwise have been lost. The therapist is in a better position to do this than the client, because far less information is evoked in the therapist than it is in the client.

Summarizing this, one may say that the therapist is taking care that no relevant information is lost for the client's processing. To do this the therapist has to keep enough distance and not be carried away by the restricted processing the client engages in spontaneously.

Previously, we stated that the therapist focuses the client's attention on relevant information that is overlooked by him. The question that arises then is: what exactly is relevant information and what is not? What is the therapist's criterion, what is the therapist

led by in selecting what he is responding to and what he will neglect? Wexler's answer to this question is that the therapist has to
select those facets which seem to refer to central aspects of the
client's functioning, or which seem unfinished; facets that seem
difficult to process. In other words: facets that appear in one way
or another significant. This betrays itself mostly in non-verbal utterances, for instance, a quivering voice, a trembling mouth, the client
suddenly changing his position, etc. . . . At that very moment, the
therapist can interrupt the client's narrative and ask something like,
'I have the feeling something in what you've just said has affected
you somehow. Can you have a closer look at it?' In this way he
can focus the client's attention on this matter.

## ii) Recalling information

A second micro-process relates to the recalling of necessary information, this is: the information associated with different facets of a
particular experience. Toukmanian calls this: facilitating the client's
recall of past experiences (1990, p. 314). Wexler and Rice call it
the evoking of meanings that are new or are lost sight of (Rice,
1974, 1984; Wexler, 1974). The therapist tries to help the client
to reconstruct past experiences as completely as possible. The
empathic response serves the function of eliciting recollection.
Evocative reflections, as described by Rice, are pre-eminently about
enlivening remembrance.

This micro-process serves two important purposes. First, it helps
the client to generate a more complete data base to further his
explorations. Secondly, it provides the therapist with the opportunity to identify those components in the client's experiences that
were inadequately processed in the past, and make sure that those
aspects are processed now. As processing now takes place on more
experiential data, the client is enabled to disrupt old restricting
schemes and replace them with new ones which enable more accurate processing of all relevant experiential data.

### iii) Organizing information

A good organization of information is one that leads to further differentiation and integration of new facets of meaning. Often, the client's own organization is inadequate in this respect, resulting in further processing either being hindered or stopped. The empathic response can facilitate further differentiation and integration of new facets of meaning.

A differentiating empathic response focuses on an important aspect of the evoked information that is not adequately elaborated on by the client himself. This response offers the client a structure that differentiates and elaborates more sharply a particular facet of meaning. Or it questions insufficiently differentiated facets of meaning so that the client will work out this facet of meaning himself. Toukmanian gives an example in which a client tells her therapist that a given situation is an emotional penalty to her. The therapist questions this expression 'emotional penalty' to get the client to clarify the meaning that this expression had for her.

An integrating empathic response tries to capture the common meaning evoked by the elements that the client is unable to synthesize at that moment. An example can help to clarify this process.

It is an example out of Wexler's 1974 article. The client, a woman who is considering leaving her husband, is discussing her relationship with him.

C1: I feel like I don't have to feel so guilty that I didn't love him. I feel like I've cared about him. But I think maybe it's good – maybe some people you can care about only so much and other people you can care about more. And I know that I can care about somebody much more than I care about him. Or else maybe I'm kidding myself. I don't know.

T1: But that's the way you feel. Like – somehow he – you can't care for him with all the caring you've got in you.

C2: That's it! And that's what I want to do. You know, care as much as I can. And I want to have somebody care about me, as much as they can.

At times the distinction between the differentiating form and the integrating form may be somewhat blurred. Sometimes an empathic response serves both functions. With clients who have a disordered mode of processing, the therapist's responses will frequently take an integrating form, since these clients will tend to elaborate on a number of different facets of meaning in experience, but be unable to attend to them and synthesize their common meaning.

For instance: A client keeps on telling stories. These stories are not linked in any way. It is up to the therapist to understand these narratives, which means that he has to understand the message in each story. The therapist must ask himself: what does the client want to communicate? It is only after the therapist has picked up the message in a story, that the client can go on with the next story. So it is important that the therapist focuses on the message, on the common meaning of each story, and not on the concrete contents.

A differentiating response is appropriate when the client tends toward premature closure in his processing, leaving significant facets of meaning unelaborated. As a result, the client fails to create change in the structure of his experiential field. The insufficient elaborating of facets of meanings is very common in therapy. So, the differentiating response is a frequently occurring intervention.


CONCLUSION

Being empathic is a process, an interaction between two persons whereby the empathizing person continuously has the willingness to tune in to the other person. This implies that the empathizing person is willing to let go of his own feeling and views. The empathically listening therapist is moving continuously and smoothly between 'appealing to himself' and 'putting himself aside'. Therefore, the therapist must function in a process-like way.

In order to come to an empathic understanding of the client, the therapist uses the various means of communication man has at his disposal: verbal and non-verbal; looking, hearing, letting resonate, talking ... and again looking, hearing, letting resonate etc. ... 'Letting resonate' then means in this context: looking inside himself for feelings, images, memories, meanings that fit in with what he is perceiving (seeing, hearing, feeling) with the client.

The empathizing therapist not only appeals to the client's cognitive capacities: his bodily feeling is involved too. He tries to be really with the other and to make real contact. In trying to get real contact with the client, the empathically listening therapist is continuously challenging the client to clarify himself, not only to the therapist, but also to himself. As such, the therapist invites the client to become more fully himself. The empathically present therapist does not merely offer the client comfort and warm understanding, balm to wounds and loneliness, but he also puts his client to work. He confronts his client with the difficult and often painful task of exploring his experiencing further. The empathizing therapist does not offer the client a 'warm nest' to bask in, but rather an understanding relationship in which the client is accepted and respected in his uniqueness on the one hand, while on the other hand there is a continuous appeal to his capacity to grow.

Research findings appear to confirm that empathy is an important therapeutic variable, particularly empathy as perceived by the client. Nevertheless, empathy research as conducted so far does not allow us to confirm Rogers' proposition that empathy is a necessary core condition for personality change as there are still a lot of questions about the construct validity of the operational definition of empathy and in most of the research only some constituent components of the empathic attitude get investigated.

Finally, I would like to say a few words on empathy-training. Being empathic is not a gift that is granted only to a few. Neither is it a technique that can be taught without commitment and involvement. It is a profound human contact capacity that can be refined. And for that purpose, training in communicative skills and working on one's own personality by means of personal therapy must be done together. In empathy-training both aspects need our attention.

I would like to end with a quotation from Rogers. In this quotation, Rogers expresses so beautifully what I hope that this discussion has evoked in all of you. He says: 'Perhaps this description makes clear that being empathic is a complex, demanding, and strong – yet also a subtle and gentle – way of being.' (Rogers, 1975, p. 4.)

REFERENCES

BARRETT-LENNARD, G. T. (1981), 'The empathy cycle: refinement of a nuclear concept', *Journal of Counseling Psychology, 28*, 91–100.

BARRETT-LENNARD, G. T. (1988), 'Listening', *Person-Centered Review, 3* (4), 410–25.

BOZARTH, J. D. (1984), 'Beyond reflection: emergent modes of empathy', in R. F. Levant and J. M. Shlien (eds.), *Client-Centered Therapy and the Person-Centered Approach: new directions in theory, research and practice* (pp. 59–75). New York: Praeger.

GENDLIN, E. T. (1968), 'The experiential response', in E. Hammer (ed.), *The Use of Interpretation in Treatment* (pp. 208–27). New York: Grune and Stratton.

GENDLIN, E. T. (1970), 'A theory of personality change', in J. T. Hart and T. M. Tomlinson (eds.), *New Directions in Client-Centered Therapy* (pp. 129–74). Boston: Houghton Mifflin.

GENDLIN, E. T. (1974), 'Client-centered and experiential psychotherapy', in D. A. Wexler and L. N. Rice (eds.), *Innovations in Client-Centered Therapy* (pp. 211–46). New York: John Wiley and Sons.

MARTIN, D. G. (1983), *Counseling and Therapy Skills*. Belmont, Ca.: Brooks and Cole.

RICE, L. N. (1974), 'The evocative function of the therapist', in D. A. Wexler and L. N. Rice (eds.), *Innovations in Client-Centered Therapy* (pp. 289–311). New York: John Wiley and Sons.

RICE, L. N. (1983), 'The relationship in client-centered therapy', in N. J. Lambert (ed.), *Psychotherapy and Patient Relationship* (pp. 36–60). Homewood: Dow Jones-Irwin.

RICE, L. N. (1984), 'Client-tasks in client-centered therapy', in R. F. Levant and J. M. Shlien (eds.), *Client-Centered Therapy and the Person-Centered Approach: new directions in theory, research and practice* (pp. 182–202). New York: Praeger.

RICE, L. N., and GREENBERG, L. S. (1990), 'Fundamental dimensions in experiential therapy: new directions in research', in G. Lietaer, J. Rombauts, and R. Van Balen (eds.), *Client-Centered and Experiential Psychotherapy in the Nineties* (pp. 397–414). Leuven: University Press.

ROGERS, C. R. (1957), 'The necessary and sufficient conditions of therapeutic personality change', *Journal of Consulting Psychology, 21*, 79–103.

ROGERS, C. R. (1975), 'Empathy: an unappreciated way of being', *The Counseling Psychologist, 5*(2), 2–10.

ROMBAUTS, J. (1984), 'Empathie: actieve ontvankelijkheid', in G. Lietaer, Ph. van Praag, and J. Swildens (eds.), *Client-Centered Psychotherapie in Beweging* (pp. 167–76). Leuven: Acco.

TOUKMANIAN, S. G. (1990), 'A schema-based information processing perspective on client change in experiential psychotherapy', in G. Lietaer, J. Rombauts and R. Van Balen (eds.), *Client-Centered and Experiential Psychotherapy in the Nineties* (pp. 309–26). Leuven: University Press.

WEXLER, D. A. (1974), 'A cognitive theory of experiencing, self-actualization, and therapeutic process', in D. A. Wexler and L. N. Rice (eds.), *Innovations in Client-Centered Therapy* (pp. 49–116). New York: J. Wiley and Sons.

## · 3 ·

# The Necessary Condition is Love: Going Beyond Self in the Person-Centred Approach

## DAVID BRAZIER

### FOREWORD

Rogers believed that 'One cannot engage in psychotherapy without giving operational evidence of an underlying . . . view of human nature' and he declared that 'It is definitely preferable . . . that such underlying views be open and explicit' (Rogers, 1957, in CRR, p. 402). This chapter is a contribution to debate about these underlying assumptions and in particular concerns itself with the extent to which human nature is envisaged as being oriented toward self or toward others. I would like to begin by inviting you to follow a line of reasoning which starts from simple considerations about therapy and goes on to question what it is that is really growth promoting. Subsequently I will elaborate the argument by approaching the same theme from other angles.

### CONSIDERATIONS ON ALTRUISM AS A THERAPEUTIC AGENT

In person-centred therapies the therapist is invited to have an unconditionally positive regard for the client (Rogers, 1961, p. 283). The therapist puts self aside in order to give full attention to the client (Rogers, 1951, p. 35). Providing accurate empathy is a thoroughly altruistic activity. Being a therapist, or indeed a helper of any description, involves 'a relationship in which at least one of the parties has the intent of promoting the growth, development, maturity, improved functioning, improved coping with life of the other' (Rogers, 1958, in CRR, p. 108).

The client's part in this endeavour is, by contrast, to focus upon self (Rogers, 1951, p. 136). The test of therapeutic effectiveness commonly assumed is whether or not the client's perception of and attitude toward self changes. The client focuses 'inwardly'. By doing so, the client makes contact with a felt sense at the edge of awareness (Gendlin, 1978). By following this 'edge' the client 'actualizes' the 'self'.

The above is familiar ground to all person-centred therapists. According to the theory of Rogers, when the therapist is able congruently to provide an ambience of unconditional positive regard expressed in the form of accurate empathy, the client will make constructive personality change (Rogers, 1957).

Now, against the background of these basic principles which specify the conditions necessary for the client to grow, the first question I wish to raise is whether the therapist also is 'self-actualizing' in the course of therapy. Rogers hypothesized that the role of client in this interaction is growth promoting, but, we may ask, is this also true for the role of therapist?

After all, if the role of therapist is not growth promoting then some further questions would arise about the wisdom of entering this profession and about the care and durability of therapists. On the other hand, if the role of therapist is growth promoting, that is, if the process is therapeutic for the therapist as well as for the client, then it would appear that this reveals another set of 'sufficient conditions' different from the ones that our theory suggests are 'necessary'.

After all, the client is probably not providing the therapist with accurate empathy nor unconditional positive regard, and in Rogers' theory the client is, by definition, incongruent. So if the therapy process is growth promoting for the therapist then we may be saying that it is growth promoting to give primary attention to someone other than self, to put one's own concerns aside and to adopt a completely altruistic stance whether or not, in the process, one receives empathy, positive regard and congruence oneself. If the conditions which apply to the client are the only ones which are growth promoting, then the self-sacrifice required of the therapist is great indeed.

One might, for the sake of completeness, try to resolve this dilemma by positing a neutral position but this does not really get us anywhere. If being a therapist is neither growth promoting nor growth negating, then the therapists would, as far as their own lives are concerned, appear to be marking time while carrying out their professional role.

Intuitively, one feels that we have to assert that the role of therapist is itself growth promoting. Insofar as Rogers himself, in his own life, may be said to have been 'self-actualizing' this was surely more by virtue of his practice as a therapist than by himself being a client. And if therefore we accept that the role of therapist is growth promoting, then, I suggest, we have to admit at least a second set of 'necessary and sufficient conditions'.

When we examine these conditions a little more closely, however, we see that perhaps the term 'conditions' is no longer quite the right term. The altruistic stance which is growth promoting is not something provided to the person from without but something generated from within.

Now let us admit a further point. Research studies have shown that while the provision of accurate empathy and so on does predispose toward good therapy outcomes, it does not guarantee them. Also, research does not reveal the means by which these conditions effect change, if indeed they do.

Also, let us take on board the fact that while it is possible to read Rogers' theory as implying a kind of determinism of the: 'if this, this and this, then that will inevitably follow' kind, it seems unlikely that Rogers intended it to be taken this way. The tone of the whole of Rogers' thinking would seem to imply freedom and responsibility rather than determinism.

Let us therefore reconsider the position of the client for a moment. The client is engaged in an encounter with a therapist who is in the flow of an altruistic way of being. If we assume that the client has some freedom in how to respond to this experience, what are the options? No doubt they are multitude but most obviously one would assume that two likely possibilities are regression and internalization or some combination of the two. In other words, clients might bathe in these benevolent conditions in a narcissistic fashion and/or they might start to take on the behaviour being so effectively modelled by the therapist (cf. Kohut, 1971). Insofar as they adopted the second option, they would, of course, themselves be beginning to fulfil our new second set of 'conditions'.

It is possible, therefore, that there is in fact only one set of conditions after all, the second set rather than the first. If this were the case, then the effectiveness of the first set would be proportional to their effectiveness in bringing the second set about and the failures of the first set would be accounted for by that proportion of clients who receive the therapist's warmth, acceptance and understanding but fail to learn to act in a similar fashion themselves.

Now, if it is actually the altruistic stance which is growth promoting rather than being in receipt of altruism, and if the value of being in receipt of it is not so much the gaining of its direct benefit but the opportunity to learn, or relearn, to adopt such a stance oneself, then our original analysis of the therapy situation takes on a different hue.

We now see that the activity of being a therapist is intrinsically growth promoting while the activity of being a client is only growth promoting insofar as the client also learns to adopt the altruistic stance. Therapy is more consistently good for therapists than it is for clients. Another important implication is that according to this new theory, unlike the original one, there is no fundamental difference between client and therapist. Both are trying to do the same thing, something which Rogers seems to have sensed intuitively but to have had difficulty formulating.

The implications of this analysis, while having a certain novelty when arrived at this way, are, of course, in accord with timeless wisdom from the world's spiritual traditions where it is widely asserted that one finds oneself in losing it.

## ROGERS ON ALTRUISM

Rogers tried to solve the problem I have just outlined in different ways. One approach was to see altruism as a way of getting one's own need for positive regard met. Thus he suggests that 'a need for positive regard . . . is universal in human beings' and the satisfaction of this need 'is reciprocal, in that when an individual discriminates himself as satisfying another's need for positive regard, he necessarily experiences satisfaction of his own need for positive regard. Hence it is rewarding both to satisfy this need in another, and to experience the satisfaction of one's own need by another' (Rogers, 1959, in CRR, p. 245). But he does not explain why or how it should be that meeting another person's need for positive regard should satisfy one's own need for it. It is by no means self-evident that this should be the case, especially so when we take on the fact that Rogers generally speaks of *unconditional* positive regard, i.e. positive regard given irrespective of whether it is returned. The word unconditional becomes meaningless if Rogers really believed that giving positive regard meant that one always received it. Rogers' theory, though well intentioned, seems incoherent in this detail if this is what he meant. Alternatively, he may have meant that the therapist who gives positive regard to another simultaneously gives positive regard to him or herself. However, this also seems inconsistent with the basic notion that the therapy process is *client*-centred.

Rogers is saying in the section just quoted that positively regarding others meets our own need for positive regard, but it is theoretically quite possible that this works the other way round as I have suggested. If we assume that our basic need is the need to love rather than the need to be loved (cf. Fromm, 1962) then the problem resolves in a more simple and straightforward way. The therapist meets this need by being a therapist and the client learns to meet this need by being directly influenced by the therapist's example.

The second way in which Rogers tried to solve this same issue was by the axiom that the self is inherently social. Thus he says:

76

'When man is less than fully man – when he denies to awareness various aspects of his experience – then indeed we have all too often reason to fear him and his behavior, as the present world situation testifies. But when he is most fully man, when he is his complete organism, when awareness of experience, that peculiarly human attribute, is most fully operating, then he is to be trusted, then his behavior is constructive. It is not always conventional. It will not always be conforming. It will be individualized. But it will also be socialized.' (Rogers, 1961, p. 106.) Now what this seems to say is that the socialized, i.e. altruistic, tendency is fundamental, and if indeed this is the case, then the theory can be more than somewhat simplified by making this the first statement rather than the last one, and making such a change would seem to have significant implications for our understanding of underlying principles and, therefore, for practice.

## PRIMARY ALTRUISM

The main suggestion of this chapter, therefore, is that our view of human nature does not have to be centred on self and the actualization of self but might, in many ways more usefully, be grounded in the idea of a need *to* love rather than a need *for* love. In Rogerian terms this would mean that we would no longer begin from an axiom that everybody has a need for positive regard but rather from an assumption that everybody has a need to provide positive regard to others.

The point here is not to refute the idea that people generally need positive regard. The argument here is not so much about what should be included in our theorizing as about what should be considered as fundamental. The intention of this chapter is to suggest the possibility that it is the altruistic orientation which is fundamental and that 'self'-development may be a derivative of this, as opposed to the commonly held notion that it is self-development which is fundamental and that the social virtues may then arise as a by-product. Changing our view of what is fundamental would,

77

nonetheless, effect a significant shift in almost all areas of our theorizing about what we do as therapists. I do not intend to explore
all these implications here, but I would like to draw attention to
some of the difficulties in existing theory which such a reorientation
might help to resolve.

## GROWTH AND DEVELOPMENT

If this thesis about intrinsic altruism is correct, then it is when this
need to give positive regard to others is frustrated that a person
declines psychologically. Frustration in life is now seen not so much
as a failure to gather narcissistic supplies, as the misfortune of living
among those who are unreceptive to one's goodwill. Without going
into great detail, this can be illustrated at different stages of the
human lifespan.

Classically, in humanistic as in psychoanalytic therapies, there
has been a tendency to assume a stage of 'primary narcissism'
(Freud, 1914) at the beginning of life and a continuing need for
'conditions of worth' (Thorne, 1992, p. 31) to be supplied to support the growing person's ego. From our new perspective, we can
see this differently. From the very first stage of life the new-born
baby has a need to look upon the mother's face. We do not need
to assume that the baby does this in order to manipulate the mother
into providing for the child. We can, with our new theory, assume
that such behaviour is intrinsically satisfying, that it is, in fact, the
first dawning of the 'other-orientation' which is intrinsic to human
nature from the very beginning.

At a slightly older age, we know that care workers are frequently
puzzled by the tenacity with which abused children continue to
believe in the virtue of their parents. The parent who abandons the
child is particularly likely to retain a special place in the child's
affections. This is very difficult to explain by a theory in which
the need to be positively regarded is fundamental, but it is easily
understood if the need to have a positive regard for others is axiomatic. No complex reasoning is necessary. The child will go on

doing what is basic to human nature and will need very compelling reasons to start doing otherwise. I suggest that the psychic injury suffered by abused children is not so much an injury to self as an injury to the possibility of continuing to regard the parent in a good light. Children will go to great lengths to try to preserve their good regard for the other, almost in spite of all odds, including taking blame for their abuse upon themselves. I am not saying that there are not other ways of explaining this type of behaviour. I am saying that the assumption of a primary need to give positive regard provides a more parsimonious, and therefore, from a scientific point of view, more satisfactory explanation.

Insofar as the person-centred approach offers a theory of human development, it hinges on the idea of conditions of worth. Since the need to be positively regarded is taken as axiomatic, satisfaction of this need is taken to be the main reinforcer in the learning process of the growing person. 'Our capacity to feel positive about ourselves is dependent upon the quality and consistency of the positive regard shown to us by others, and where this has been selective (as to some degree it must be for all of us) we are victims of what Rogers described as *conditions of worth*' (Thorne, 1992, p. 31). However, with our new hypothesis, we are led to ask again why it is that the parent's smile is reinforcing for the child. The old theory suggests that the child pleases the parent in order to receive the parent's positive regard, whereas the new theory suggests that the child simply wants the parent to be pleased. We do not have to assume any deviousness on the part of the child.

At the other end of the lifespan, we similarly know that elderly people lose heart when they believe they are no longer useful. With our new theory, we do not have to assume that the desire to be useful is due to 'conditioning' nor that people are serving a neurotic need by wanting to retain a role which is beneficial to others. We can simply accept it at face value as the normal and healthy human response.

The human being is intrinsically outward-looking and a positive life is one in which this outward gaze is permitted to be positive. In midlife, relationships which turn sour do so not so much because one or both partners fail to get all the love they need but because the love they give is not received.

How then does the ego evolve? I suggest that the ego evolves out of the repertoire of strategies which the child evolves to try to maintain the primary altruistic stance in the face of aspects of the world which prove unreceptive. Here, in a sense, we are reversing the theory of Kohut (1971). With him, our theory suggests that character develops as a consequence of disappointments. These disappointments are, however, now to be seen not so much as failures in the perfect empathy of the parent as situations in which the child must use ingenuity to hold on to the positive stance. Throughout life people struggle to maintain a positive view in the face of discouraging information. The theory presented here adds a new twist to Freud's famous comment that 'we are bound to fall ill if, in consequence of frustration, we are unable to love' (Freud, 1914, p. 78).

Taylor (1989) has gathered together a wealth of research data to refute the idea that depression is the product of an unrealistic view of the world. Actually it is the mentally healthy who maintain a view which is more positive than the facts can justify. It is human nature to look on the bright side.

So if the disappointment is not too great, the child will 'get over it'. The negative information will be accepted and integrated into the positive regard repertoire. This collection of strategies, I submit, constitutes the ego. The ego thus becomes the stock of means which the person holds by which a positive view of life may be restored in adverse circumstances. The more varied and versatile the stock, the more character strength we say the person possesses. Maturity is the capacity to meet adversity, to remain dignified in undignified circumstances and to stay in good morale even when the most serious obstacles are put in the way of one's basic need to see others positively and to see the world as a good place. In passing, we could note that religious faith provides an example of a well-developed version of such a repertoire.

We do know that many of the clients we see suffer greatly from a negative view of themselves and from a sense of guilt and that this has its roots in earlier life experience. Why should this be so common? If the basic need of the growing person is to be positively regarded, why would a lack of such regard give rise to feelings of guilt on the part of the child? With our new theory, however, we see that the problem for the child is not so much one of trying to get the good regard of the parent but one of trying to sustain a positive view of the parent. Taking blame upon oneself is one possible strategy for achieving this. It appears that one may well take the blame upon oneself in order to be able to sustain a positive regard for the other. Positive self-regard may be sacrificed if this is necessary to maintain the more fundamental need to regard the other positively. So children are simply following their basic nature in taking the blame upon themselves. It may not be just, but it is easily understandable in terms of our new theory.

The examples sketched here show that, if adopted, the basic proposition of this chapter would stand a good deal of our present theorizing on its head. Many of the lines of reasoning which are commonly used to show how socialized behaviour can be reduced to selfish motivation would be reversed and therapists would, I suggest, listen to their clients with a different ear. The function of therapy can be seen, in the light of this principle, to consist in providing a situation where the client can return to natural, altruistic functioning. In the therapy situation, the client sees the therapist being attentive and, at a deep level, is reminded of a way of living which is not turned in upon self.

Since this suggestion is rather radical, I propose now to look at the related area of self theory in order to consider the question from the other side, as it were.

SELF THEORY

Given that there is at least room for discussion about whether it is self-regard or regard for others which is therapeutic and growth promoting, it may be interesting to take a digression into the question of what is meant by self in the first place.

81

When we turn to this field, it is quickly apparent that the term self, and its variants such as ego, are so variously used by different theorists that it is often hard to make useful comparisons between them. The bipolar self of Kohut, the transcendental ego of Husserl, the organismic self of Rogers, the ich, es and uber-ich of Freud have only very approximate equivalence of meaning. For Jung, the journey of life is a progression from the ego to the self (Stevens, 1990). In Buddhism, ego and self are synonyms and both are regarded as pernicious (e.g. Gyatso, 1986, pp. 264–82). In humanistic psychology we are told to love ourselves. In traditional Christianity the self is something to be mortified (Thomas à Kempis, *The Imitation of Christ*, ch. 3), yet we are also enjoined to 'love thy neighbour as thy *self*' (Matt. 19.19). The term ego is generally thought of as deriving from Freud but it actually derives from his translators since he himself only spoke of 'das Ich' (= the I); 'The term "self" (Das Selbst) occurs only very rarely in Freud's work' (McIntosh, 1986). Language is so confused that it is often hard to know whether two theorists are in agreement or in opposition to one another. The 'present muddle' (Redfearn, 1983, p. 102), where 'The terms "ego" and "self" . . . are . . . in some cases used one way and sometimes in exactly the opposite way' (ibid. p. 105), derives in part from the proliferation of different psychological schools but, more fundamentally from the enigmatic nature of the topic.

The matter is complicated even in common speech where the word 'self' has at least two quite separate usages, viz. as a noun and as a reflexive pronoun, which are nonetheless easily confused. When I say that my computer printer is 'self-feeding' I am not implying that it has a soul or psyche, but when we talk about self-love it is unclear whether we are talking about devotion to a transcendent principle at the essence of our being, or referring to indulgence in more than our share of chocolate cake or making an oblique reference to masturbation.

When we come to terms like 'self-concept' and 'self-regard', we are, therefore, in something of a minefield. Thus for some people at least the concept of self is likely to include the idea of something unchanging. In this conception, self is that which endures through the flux of life, and we can see that this notion is associated with the traditional idea of an immortal soul. Clearly this is not the self-concept which Rogers had in mind when he wrote: 'The individual has within himself or herself vast resources for self-understanding, for altering his or her self-concept, attitudes and self-directed behavior' (CCR, p. 135). That which endures is not that which can be changed, though even here 'self' and 'self-concept' are probably not to be equated. On the other hand there is at least an implication in this statement by Rogers that the self-concept is something which changes from time to time rather than continuously, but he may well not have thought this to be the case for the self itself, if you still follow me.

In the tradition of Rogers we distinguish the 'self-concept' from the experiencing or 'organismic-self'. Whether the latter is equivalent to what analysts refer to as the unconscious is a moot point. Whether either is an active agent capable of being a subject in the behaviour of the person rather than simply an object or construct of perception, is also unclear.

These enigmas draw attention to a basic dilemma for any therapy which aims at consciousness as a goal. This is as follows. Consciousness is always consciousness of an object. 'In ordinary, everyday conduct, we forget about our "selves"' (Murakami, 1990, p. 3), but even in reflective contemplation, it is impossible to be conscious of the subject of consciousness. The subject of consciousness *can* be objectified and looked at but by the time this has been done it has ceased to be the subject and has become an object. To repeat in simpler language: I can perceive objects. Consciousness consists of perception of objects. The 'I' can be considered as an object and perceived. When the 'I' is being considered as an object and perceived, there must be another (subject) I perceiving it. The perceiving I is not knowable directly. It is therefore in the nature of the situation that we are always perceiving an 'other' even when we think we are perceiving ourselves. Even the self we see has to be objectified to be seen. A fully functioning person, we may say, is one looking at objects, not one really looking at self. A person is intrinsically outward-looking.

There is, therefore, a void at the centre of our being as far as experience is concerned because whatever the term 'centre of our being' may mean, it denotes the notional point from which perception occurs, a point which can, therefore, never itself be in the line of sight. This idea of a void at the centre of things feels uncomfortable at first but is in line with much other modern thinking where even galaxies are now conceived to be vortices around an empty centre.

We are intrinsically organized to focus outside of self. We can only have a notion of self by making self something which is outside of self; that is by making it into an other. Self is something notional rather than something which can be encountered.

The natural functioning of the person is other-oriented and not self-oriented. It can only be self-oriented by making self into an other first. Such a 'self-as-other' is a 'self-concept' all right but it is not the self-itself, nor could it ever be. The idea that the self-concept coincides with the self-itself rests upon the idea that the self stays constant during the procedure of objectification but this seems most implausible.

If the natural functioning of the person is other-oriented, it seems that what would be therapeutic might be to help people remain in or return to this condition. This is, of course, rather different from what most therapists conceive themselves to be doing.

Rogers tells us that 'the way that the person looks at him or herself is the most important factor in predicting future behavior' (Rogers, 1986, in CRR, p. 209). But the self which is looked at cannot be the same self as the self which is looking. The objectification process may be a deduction from direct personal experience or it may be filtered through the perceptions of others (cf. James, 1890). Thus one might think oneself a sickly person because one had noticed the frequency of bodily pains or one might think oneself a worthwhile person because one had listened to one's admirers. Either way, it is clear enough that the self-concept is exactly that, a concept. It is a construct built up from clues, not something directly perceived. There is thus a certain degree of arbitrariness about it. Indeed, it is perfectly possible to have a multitude of different self-concepts (Rowan, 1990).

In contrast to Rogers' statement we might suggest that it is the way that a person looks at others which is the most important factor in predicting future behaviour, and it can be argued that this latter assertion is of wider application. There are plenty of people who, when asked what they think of themselves, have very little idea, and there are some who would not even initially know what they were being asked. There are, however, no people who cannot immediately say something about how they regard others, excepting, of course, those who may be under some coercion to remain silent. The way that a person regards him or herself, if indeed they do, is a derivative of the way they regard others, not the other way round.

Regarding others is a natural activity. Regarding self is an art which must be learned and requires some sophistication. It is less fundamentally a part of human nature.

In modern societies, each of us is required to have one or more self-concepts and, in certain social situations, to be willing to display or defend them. Paradoxically, it does appear to me that the self-concept exists, not so much to assist self-actualization as to effect social control. This finds concrete form in the fact that we commonly have to carry documents to say who we are. Self-regard is a social artefact rather than a personal one. Other-regard is human nature.

Although we are required by society to have a self-concept, what is most personal and satisfying are those situations where we do not have to be remembering who we are. These are situations where we find intimacy, spontaneity and concern for others and for the natural environment. One is perhaps most alive when one feels moved by another or in direct communion with nature and most real when one is engaged in some action of evident intrinsic value.

On the other hand, when one has been engaged in self-directed activities for a time, a sense of unreality and alienation becomes apparent. The most opulent and pampered members of society who have everything self could require give little evidence of being the most happy, and the person who lives in a world which is almost wholly made up of self-projections we declare to be mad and see as one most to be pitied. When people reach a condition in which they only consume care and no longer provide it to others, a sense of meaninglessness sets in and this is frequently fatal. None of these phenomena are straightforwardly explained by a theory which takes self-regard as its first principle but they are all quite obvious if we assume that other-regard is primary.

My suggestion, therefore, is that consciousness has nothing much to do with self-concern and rather more to do with self-forgetting. From this point of view, 'self-actualization' is a rather unfortunate term. The fully functioning person does not create something unitary called a self. He or she is too totally immersed in life for that. The fully functioning person 'is a being in the moment, with little self-conscious awareness' (Rogers, 1961, p. 147). This is the point where 'Self as an object tends to disappear' (ibid.).

A certain strength of character emerges from experience through the attempt to maintain the primary altruism through the adversities of life and if we need a collective noun for the repertoire of strategies which make up such versatility, then we might call this the self or ego but, in this analysis at least, this is clearly a secondary phenomenon rather than the basic grounding of our theory and, in any case, the more old-fashioned term 'character' might be more apt.

## THE SELF, ORGANISMIC AND CONCEPTUAL

Rogers clearly believed that a definition of mental health included some degree of convergence between experience, self and ideal self (Rogers, 1959, in CRR, p. 242). Self here again seems to refer to self-concept. In other words, we are healthy when what we experience coincides with what we believe we are, and when this in turn coincides with what we would like to be. Now the least malleable of these three is presumably experience, so health is defined in terms of bringing self-concept and self-ideal into line with experience rather than the other way about. Hence, we have pride of place given to the organismic self: 'psychotherapy is a process whereby man becomes his organism' (Rogers, 1961, p. 103) and we have therapy defined in terms of bringing the client closer to experience: 'Therapy seems to mean a getting back to basic sensory and visceral experience' (Rogers, 1961, p. 103). It follows, however, fairly readily from this that in the healthy state so defined, self-concept must be in a state of flux since this is the case with experience.

It also follows, since experience is always experience *of* something, that by giving primacy to the organismic self, Rogers is actually breaking down the self-object boundary, and doing so in a direction which ensures that the self will become immersed in the other rather than vice versa.

As already said, it is very easy to become confused in interpreting this literature because we commonly use terms inconsistently. When the term self is used, most people have a notion of something which either does not change or only changes slowly. Organismic experience, on the other hand, is a flux. The now commonly used term 'organismic self' therefore equates something which in the common mind is rather solid and enduring (my self) with something which is rather fluid and mercurial (the flow of experience). It joins, as it were, a solid and a liquid in a single entity. It does seem that in Rogers' conception, if we may stay with this analogy, it is the solid that is dissolved in the liquid rather than the liquid which is contained by or absorbed into the solid.

So, person-centred therapies give pride of place to the organismic self and aim to bring self-concept into line with experience, even though the line is a moving one. And experience, in Rogers' conception, very largely means perception.

The whole philosophical movement called phenomenology, which seems to have influenced Rogers considerably, is an attempt to get to grips with the notion that perception is the leader of the human dance. And perception, of course, is always perception of something. Rogers' practical aim in psychotherapy is primarily to understand the client's perception. He says, 'I am *not* trying to "reflect feelings". I am trying to determine whether my understanding of the client's inner world is correct – whether I am seeing it as he or she is experiencing it at this moment' (Rogers, 1986, in CRR, p. 128). The inclusion of the words 'at this moment' to me indicate Rogers' awareness that what he is talking about is something which is in constant flux.

In summary, therefore, the term self is unclear both in its meaning and in its usefulness. It is not clear what self-awareness is. It is not possible that it means knowledge of the knower, as it were. It could be knowledge of a construct called the 'self-concept' but it is unclear what such a construct refers to in the 'real world'. It could be awareness of the flux of experience, and Rogers sometimes seems to want it to be this, but this is quite different from what most people seem to mean when they talk about knowing oneself. And if it is equated with the perception of the flux of experience then this is actually an assertion that in our deepest nature we are outward-looking. It would appear, in fact, that the word 'self' refers to many different things, and, sometimes, may not even refer to anything at all, and this does not provide a very firm base for theory or practice. Most of the time, and especially when engaged in anything worthwhile, people are not primarily focused on self but upon 'objects' and self has to be made into an object in order to be focused upon but any such conceptualization gives it a degree of fixity which Rogers repeatedly points out belies its real fluid nature.

Sheldon Kopp popularized a saying: 'If you meet the Buddha on the road, kill him.' What this phrase means is not, as is often thought, that no one can teach you anything, but rather that if you think you see your actualized self (i.e. your Buddha), you are mistaken. I suggest, the therapist is most 'self-actualizing', if we may use this term to mean most fully in accord with his or her nature, when fully engaged in the other-directed, that is altruistic, activity of genuine unconditional positive regard and expresses this in empathy for the other. Self-actualization occurs when self is forgotten. Clients, on the other hand, are incongruent precisely in the extent to which self-preoccupation has distracted them from the world of others to whom they need to attend. If we could realize that the self-concept is an 'object' in our world, just like others, we would no doubt realize that there is no particular reason to give it pride of place in our attentions. The whole point of a client-centred therapy is that it is to do with helping others, but if we believe that helping others is a good idea we must believe that it is a good idea for the client as well as for ourselves and not try to put ourselves on a different plane from those we help.

The contention of this chapter, therefore, is not so much to exclude other views as to say that it seems simpler, more parsimonious, to take the need to love as axiomatic rather than to take the need to be loved as fundamental and to argue that this is also more consistent with the phenomenological roots of our approach and with the basic facts of human nature as we encounter them daily.

I do not here spell out practice implications of such a shift of theory. I do believe that a change of the therapist's outlook affects practice but spelling out the intricacies of this would be work for another paper. By way of illustration, I can say that I often find it easier to empathize with a client when I do not seek to reduce such statements as 'I didn't want to hurt him' to a supposedly more fundamental selfish motive and when I do stay open to the possibility that forgiving someone who has wronged one may be just as or even more therapeutic than becoming angrily assertive (cf. Canale, 1990). Many clients who tell me about how they have been harmed by their parents, seem nonetheless to be still longing to love them and, with the help of the theory outlined here, I find this easier to empathize with. When they can find a route to reconciliation this seems to provide the most satisfactory outcome. When they consolidate their anger, the gains in morale seem very temporary.

Before finishing, I would like to draw attention to one other implication. This has to do with the training of therapists. I am a strong believer in the idea that the therapist must have made some progress in life and that personal therapy should play a part in this. Students at my own institute are required to be in therapy themselves for some part of their training. I was therefore somewhat taken aback by Wheeler's (1991) recent review of research which suggests that being in therapy at best makes no difference to a person's ability to be a therapist and, in some cases, may actually make trainees into worse therapists. This perhaps was one of those disappointments that make one grow a bit. My hunch now, and it is no more than a hunch at this stage, is that not a little of the therapy which is provided these days does indeed encourage the client toward a more self-oriented way of being and this may be especially the case where the 'client' is actually a trainee therapist. The prevailing ethos of many 'growth' activities these days is one of adulation for self-seeking attitudes and this may not be productive.

## CONCLUSION

Therapy is an altruistic activity. If we believe in it then we must believe that such altruism is healthy. If it is healthy for the therapist it is healthy for the client. Rogers asserts that the person is social in basic nature but still bases his theory upon the idea of a need to receive positive regard and upon a concept of self which may now be becoming outdated (Holdstock, see chapter 12). Contemporary Western psychological theory generally is self-oriented but much of the theory of self is incoherent. An alternative basis for theory is provided by the notion of a primary altruism rather than a primary narcissism, at the root of human nature. This provides a more direct explanation of many phenomena which are difficult to explain by other current theories. Adopting this new hypothesis reverses many common lines of logic in psychology and has implications for theory building, for practice and for training.

REFERENCES

CANALE, J. R. (1990), 'Altruism and forgiveness as therapeutic agents in psychotherapy', *Journal of Religion and Health*, 29, 4, pp. 297–301.
FREUD, S. (1914), 'On narcissism: an introduction', in Strachey J.

(trans.), Richards, A. (ed.), *On Metapsychology*, Penguin Freud Library, volume 11. London: Penguin Books, pp. 65–97.

FROMM, E. (1962), *The Art of Loving*. London: Unwin.

GENDLIN, E. T. (1978), *Focusing*. New York: Bantam.

GYATSO, K. (1986), *Meaningful to Behold*. London: Tharpa.

JAMES, W. (1890/1950), *Principles of Psychology*. Cambridge, Ma: Harvard University Press.

KOHUT, H. (1971), *The Analysis of the Self*. London: Hogarth.

MCINTOSH, D. (1986), 'The ego and the self in the thought of Sigmund Freud', *International Journal of Psychoanalysis*, 67, pp. 429–48.

MURAKAMI, Y. (1990), 'Two types of civilization: transcendental and hermeneutic', *Japan Review*, 1, pp. 1–34.

REDFEARN, J. W. T. (1983), 'Ego and self: terminology', *Journal of Analytical Psychology*, 28, pp. 91–106.

ROGERS, C. R. (1951), *Client-Centred Therapy*. London: Constable.

ROGERS, C. R. (1957), 'The necessary and sufficient conditions of therapeutic personality change', *Journal of Counselling Psychology*, 21, 2, pp. 95–103.

ROGERS, C. R. (1961), *On Becoming a Person*. London: Constable.

ROWAN, J. (1990), *Subpersonalities*. London: Routledge.

STEVENS, A. (1990), *On Jung*. London: Routledge.

TAYLOR, S. E. (1989), *Positive Illusions: creative self-deception and the healthy mind*. New York: Basic Books.

THORNE, B. (1992), *Carl Rogers*. London: Sage.

WHEELER, S. (1991), 'Personal therapy: an essential aspect of counsellor training or a distraction from focusing upon the client', *International Journal for the Advancement of Counselling*, 14, pp. 193–202.

## Abbreviation

CRR: *The Carl Rogers Reader*, edited by H. Kirschenbaum and V. L. Henderson. London: Constable (1990).

## · 4 ·

# Not Necessarily Necessary but Always Sufficient

## JEROLD BOZARTH

It was thirty years ago that Carl Rogers (1957) postulated the psychological conditions that he viewed as necessary and sufficient to bring about therapeutic personality change. This statement consisted of a series of hypotheses meant to clarify and extend knowledge in the field of psychotherapy and, as well, in other kinds of relationships.

Considerable attention was given to these hypotheses between 1957 and 1987. This attention included:

1. A de-emphasis on techniques and methods identified with client-centred therapy; i.e. 'The conditions apply to any situation in which constructive personality change occurs, whether we are thinking of classical psychoanalysis or any of its modern offshoots, or Adlerian Therapy, or any others.' (Rogers, 1957, p. 101.)

2. Conceptualizations that were operationally defined for measurement instruments (Barrett-Lennard, 1962; Rogers, Gendlin, Kiesler and Traux, 1967; Traux and Carkhuff, 1967) and subsequently developed to train therapists with emphasis on systematic training programmes (Carkhuff, 1969; Gordon, 1970, 1976).

3. A host of studies that, during the 1960s, resulted in the conclusion of Traux and Mitchell (1971) that the attitudinal qualities as hypothesized by Rogers and determined via research reports were *necessary and sufficient*.

4. An increasingly accepted statement that occurred prior to the

1970s that the conditions were *necessary but not sufficient*. This conclusion later received credence in reviews of the research (e.g. Parloff, Waskow and Wolfe, 1978).

At this point, psychological literature continued to extend the view that the conditions were *necessary but not sufficient* as authors used varied explanatory schemes in their reviews (Gelso and Carter, 1985; Orlinsky and Howard, 1987).

The remainder of this chapter examines the substance of this conclusion (i.e. that the conditions are necessary but not sufficient) from the perspectives of the research results, relevant literature, and the theoretical foundation of the person-centred approach. It will be concluded that this deviation has little, if any, substantial validation. It will be concluded that, rather than the conditions being necessary but not sufficient, it is more plausible to consider the conditions as not necessarily necessary but always sufficient.

## THE NECESSARY AND SUFFICIENT CONDITIONS

Rogers postulated that, if six conditions existed over a period of time, no other conditions are necessary and these conditions are sufficient to induce constructive personality change. These conditions stated by Rogers (1957) are:

1. Two persons are in psychological contact.
2. The first, whom we shall term the client, is in a state of incongruence, being vulnerable or anxious.
3. The second person, whom we shall term the therapist, is congruent or integrated in the relationship.
4. The therapist experiences unconditional positive regard for the client.
5. The therapist experiences an empathic understanding of the client's internal frame of reference and endeavours to communicate this experience to the client.
6. The communication to the client of the therapist's empathic

understanding and unconditional positive regard is to a minimal degree achieved.

No other conditions are necessary. If these six conditions exist, and continue over a period of time, this is sufficient. The process of constructive personality change will follow (p. 96).

## RESEARCH EVIDENCE

The research generated by Rogers' hypotheses has followed several general patterns.

*1950–1960*: Research results predominantly conducted and reported by investigators from the University of Chicago supported the speculation that the conditions were necessary and sufficient for therapeutic personality change (Cartwright, 1957; Chordoroff, 1954; Rogers, 1959; Rogers and Diamond, 1954; Seeman and Raskin, 1953).

*1960–1970*: The research results over this period are summarized by Traux and Mitchell (1971) as supporting the necessity and sufficiency of the conditions. Their review of the literature found that higher levels of the conditions were related to positive outcomes. Clients of therapists measured at higher levels on the conditions improved significantly more than did clients of therapists measured at lower levels of the conditions.

*1970–1980*: The research continued to focus upon the relationships of the attitudinal conditions to client outcome. The most general conclusions were that: 1. 'More complex relationships exist among therapist, patients, and techniques' (Parloff, Waskow and Wolfe, 1978, p. 273); 2. 'Such relationship dimensions are rarely sufficient for patient change' (Gurman, 1977, p. 503); and 3. 'Our conclusion must be that the relationship between the interpersonal skills and client outcome has not been investigated and, consequently, nothing definitive can be said about the relative efficacy of high and low levels of empathy, warmth, and genuineness' (Mitchell, Bozarth and Krauft, 1977, p. 488).

*1980–1987*: The research direction moved away from Rogers' hypotheses to examine facets of therapy in different ways (Gelso and Carter, 1985; Orlinsky and Howard, 1987). Gelso and Carter noted that from their perspective (i.e. psychoanalytic) 'the conditions originally specified by Rogers are neither necessary nor sufficient although it seems clear that such conditions are facilitative' (p. 220). However, Patterson (1984; 1985) challenged recent research summaries, considering them to be unsubstantiated conclusions of research. Patterson believes that the inherent bias of the reviews generally distorts the accuracy and meaning of the research summaries.

It should also be noted that research in Europe on the attitudinal qualities has supported the notion that the conditions are necessary and sufficient (Tausch, 1978; 1987a). However, Tausch (1982) has also reported other activities as being helpful to various individuals and pointed to convergencies with behaviour therapy (Tausch, 1987b).

Several authors (Bozarth, 1983; Mitchell, Bozarth and Krauft, 1977; and Watson, 1984) have suggested that the conditions have not been adequately tested. Mitchell *et al.* report that the absolute levels of the conditions for groups of 'higher' functioning therapists are so seldom high that the notion that they are in the experimental group as higher functioning therapists does not lend credence to the research results. They note, 'Under such circumstances, it seems to us virtually impossible to explore the full impact of empathy, warmth, and genuineness on client change' (p. 498).

Bozarth (1983) suggests that therapist samples so seldom include individuals who hold the basic philosophy of the client-centred/person-centred approach that research results on the conditions are thoroughly confounded.

Watson (1984) views Rogers' (1957) statements as tenets in a scientific method experiment and suggests that they have never been scientifically investigated because several of the six tenets have been ignored.

*In summary*, the research summaries of the evidence regarding the relationship of the attitudinal qualities to client improvement fundamentally disagree. Patterson (1984; 1985) and Bergin and Lambert (1978) summarize the research as supportive of Rogers' hypotheses while others noted by Parloff, Waskow and Wolfe (1978) are critical of the positive research results. Others (Bozarth, 1983; Mitchell, Bozarth and Krauft, 1977; and Watson, 1984) question the extent to which the hypotheses have been investigated. Nearly all investigations examine the relationships of the levels of the attitudinal qualities to process or outcome measures. Seldom are other treatment procedures compared in a way that the necessity and sufficiency of the conditions can be investigated.

It is noteworthy for the purpose of this chapter that there is virtually no research that supports the position that the attitudinal qualities are *necessary but not sufficient* for therapeutic personality change. The research summaries often disagree. There are no direct research inquiries concerning this question.

## RELEVANT LITERATURE

A survey of the literature does not provide a definitive beginning of the first references to the belief that the conditions are necessary but not sufficient.

Ellis (1959), responding to the requisite conditions to basic personality change, stated his view that there are probably no absolute conditions for constructive personality change. However, the statement that seems to be the forerunner for the 'necessary but not sufficient' statement was Krumboltz's (1967) reference to 'The Necessary But Insufficient Skill of Empathic Understanding' (p. 224). He referred to the skill of empathic listening as being 'only one of the many skills which a behaviorally oriented counselor must learn' (p. 224). He viewed empathic listening as the *sine qua non* of client-centred counselling. He pointed out that this view does not fit the behavioural model since, among other things, the behavioural counsellor must learn how to translate client-presented problems into achievable objectives.

This behavioural context continued with the proposal of action dimensions (Patterson, 1969; Traux and Carkhuff, 1967; Carkhuff, 1969) that reasserted the therapist as an agent who should direct client behaviour towards more effective functioning.

It is ironic that models developed from Rogers' conceptualizations (Traux and Carkhuff, 1967; Carkhuff, 1969) incorporated elements that encourage therapist interventions. Eventually, the models presented the client-centred component as the initial but incomplete effort because clients had to be encouraged toward action dimensions. It is primarily this model combined with the trend of the psychological literature toward cognitive behaviourism that concludes that the conditions are necessary but not sufficient. It seems that most authors of the psychotherapeutic literature (as well as authors of research reviews) do not understand or accept the supposition that the client knows best about his or her life and improves that life when an atmosphere is provided by a therapist who operates on this premise. It seems that the authors cannot discard the belief that the therapist must intervene in some way, at some point, to set the client in an appropriate direction. This presupposition can only lead to the conclusion that the conditions are not sufficient. It is a predetermined conclusion that ignores one of the fundamental premises of the person-centred approach, i.e. that it is the client who knows best what hurts, what direction to go, and that the client has vast resources for self-renewal. In Rogers' (1961) words:

> It is the client who knows what hurts, what directions to go, what problems are crucial, what problems have been deeply buried. It began to occur to me that unless I had a need to demonstrate my own cleverness and learning, I would do better to rely on the client for the direction of movement in the process. (p. 12.)

The bulk of the psychological literature simply examines Rogers' conceptualizations from frames of reference that are markedly different from Rogers' contentions. As such, no conclusion could possibly be reached that would threaten the interventive views of therapists.

The remainder of this chapter discusses the conceptualization of the necessary and sufficient conditions within the framework of person-centred theory.

## THEORETICAL FOUNDATIONS

This section reviews the theoretical foundation of the client-centred/person-centred approach in relation to the hypotheses of the 'necessary and sufficient conditions for therapeutic personality change'. I have offered a summary of the approach with the following statement.

> It is when the therapist can embody the attitudinal qualities of congruency, unconditional positive regard, and empathic understanding in the therapeutic relationship with the client in a way that the client can perceive/experience these qualities with the locus of control belonging to the client then the actualizing process of the client is promoted. (Bozarth, 1987.)

Therapeutic personality change occurs as the individual's actualizing process is promoted.

As noted previously, the conclusions in the literature that the conditions are not sufficient are views from other frames of reference (e.g. behavioural, psychoanalytic) which do not consider the assumption of the actualizing tendency. Alternative assumptions have a predominant set that does not accept self-sufficient development as a result of the presence and communication of the attitudinal qualities of the therapist. The therapist from these views is predisposed to act or intervene to influence the client. Rogers' (1980) central point that we are tapping into a tendency which permeates all organic life is simply not considered in such presentations. Thus, Krumboltz (1969) cannot accept empathic understanding, which he describes (somewhat inaccurately) as the *sine qua non* of Rogerian therapy, because it does not fit the behavioural paradigm. Likewise, proponents of Human Relations Training

Models (Egan, 1982; Carkhuff, 1969), acting on the premise that one must go beyond the client-centred approach since client-centred therapists seldom get to action (Carkhuff, 1981), either do not understand or do not accept the basic foundation of the client-centred/person-centred approach, i.e. the actualizing tendency.

A brief re-examination of Rogers' statement that the conditions are necessary and sufficient is essential at this point. Rogers (1957) states: 'No other conditions are necessary. If these six conditions exist, and continue over a period of time, this is sufficient. The process of constructive personality change will follow.' (p. 96.) The implication of the theory is that the consistent existence and communication of the six conditions foster and promote the actualizing tendency of an individual in a process that includes constructive personality change.

The fact of the matter is that the necessity and sufficiency of the conditions are valid in terms of (in fact, are part of) the theoretical framework. Changes concerning the statement to necessary but not sufficient from other theoretical frameworks have no validity. It simply means, in cyclical conundrum, that the conditions are not viewed as sufficient within different theoretical frameworks. The validity of statements is dependent upon scientific inquiry (Seeman, 1987) and not upon different theoretical positions.

The conclusion that the conditions are necessary but not sufficient is, as noted earlier, not supported by scientific inquiry, and only supported in the literature by those who hold different theoretical stances. Of course, Rogers' postulation that the conditions are sufficient as they apply to any situation can likewise only be investigated through scientific inquiry as he meant it to be. It is noteworthy that Rogers' theoretical statement is viewed from the perceptual stance of the therapist. He speculated that, if the therapist could *experience* unconditional positive regard and empathic understanding and *endeavour to communicate* this experience, and if these *therapist experiences* were to a minimal degree received by the client, then the process of change would follow. If these circumstances exist over a period of time, he presumes that the other theoretical frames of reference do not matter to (and will not interfere with?) these conditions. *If these conditions exist, no other conditions are necessary. They are sufficient.* It is significant that this statement is theoretically consistent. In linear terms: If the conditions exist over time then nothing else is necessary and the conditions are sufficient. Rogers does not talk about whether or not there might be other factors sufficient to induce therapeutic personality change other than to state his hypothesis that significant positive personality change always occurs in a relationship. It is interesting, however, that he identifies conditions 2 and 6 as: 'the characteristics of the relationship which are regarded as essential by defining the necessary characteristics of each person in the relationship' (p. 96). These conditions state that one person is in a state of incongruence and the other communicates the experience of these conditions in a way that, at least, is minimally achieved. There is, however, a baffling question: Can a vulnerable person experience the conditions when they are not provided by the particular person of the therapist? Is it possible that the vulnerable person's (e.g. the client's) actualizing process can be promoted in other ways? It seems to me theoretically consistent and functionally true that people do improve therapeutically without being in relationship with therapists who consistently hold these attitudes.

I am at this point raising the question: Are the conditions not necessarily necessary? I believe this is a useful secondary inquiry because it might remind us of the remarkable resilience of human beings who, in my opinion, quite often overcome intolerable circumstances (and sometimes their therapists) to improve. This view is predicated on the concept of the actualizing tendency which is the foundation block (Rogers, 1980) of the person-centred approach. The actualizing tendency is described as the central source of energy in the human organism. Rogers' (1980) conceptualization is that of 'a tendency toward fulfilment, toward actualization, involving not only maintenance but also the enhancement of the organism' (p. 123). Humans are *always* doing the best they can with a 'flow of movement toward constructive fulfilment of its inherent possibilities' (Rogers, 1980, p. 117). One of Rogers' (1980) metaphors aptly captures this process:

The actualizing tendency can, of course, be thwarted or warped, but it cannot be destroyed without destroying the organism. I remember that in my boyhood, the bin in which we stored our winter's supply of potatoes was in the basement, several feet below a small window. The conditions were unfavorable, but the potatoes would begin to sprout pale white sprouts, so unlike the healthy green shoots they sent up when planted in the soil in the spring. But these sad, spindly sprouts would grow 2 or 3 feet in length as they reached toward the distant light of the window. The sprouts were, in their bizarre, futile growth, a sort of desperate expression of the directional tendency I have been describing. They would never become plants, never mature, never fulfill their real potential. But under the most adverse circumstances, they were striving to become. Life would not give up, even if it could not flourish. In dealing with clients whose lives have been terribly warped, in working with men and women on the back wards of state hospitals, I often think of those potato sprouts. So unfavorable have been the conditions in which these people have developed that their lives often seem abnormal, twisted, scarcely human. Yet, the directional tendency in them can be trusted. The clue to understanding their behavior is that they are striving, in the only ways that they perceive as available to them, to move toward growth, toward becoming. To healthy persons, the results may seem bizarre and futile, but they are life's desperate attempt to become itself. This potent constructive tendency is an underlying basis of the person-centered approach. (pp. 118–19.)

One of the aspects of this metaphor is that the sprouts of the potatoes move toward the distant light. They seek growth-inducive conditions! It seems conceivable that individuals also seek and use whatever is available to them for constructive change. There are certainly individuals who report significant felt change and improved function from experiencing a religious conversion, a sunset, a smile, a traumatic experience, and so on. The remarkable resilience of humans in terms of the actualizing tendency leads me to conclude that the conditions may not necessarily be necessary.

*In summary*, this chapter challenges recent conclusions of research reviews and the psychological literature that the conditions postulated by Rogers as necessary and sufficient for therapeutic personality change are necessary but not sufficient.

Examination of recent reviews of research, relevant literature, and the theoretical underpinnings of the person-centred approach leads to the conclusion that there is no substantial evidence to refute Rogers' position. Further consideration of the theoretical underpinnings suggests to me that, rather than conclude the conditions are *necessary but not sufficient*, it is more accurate to conclude that the conditions are *not necessarily necessary but always sufficient*.

## REFERENCES

BARRETT-LENNARD, G. T. (1962), 'Dimensions of therapist responses as causal factors in therapeutic change', *Psychological Monographs*, 65 (43, Whole No: 562).

BERGIN, A. E., and LAMBERT, M. J. (1978), 'The evaluation of therapeutic outcomes', in S. L. Garfield and A. E. Bergin (eds.), *Handbook of Psychotherapy and Behavior Change: an empirical analysis* (2nd ed.). New York: John Wiley and Sons.

BOZARTH, J. D. (1983), 'Current research on client-centered therapy in the USA', in M. Wolf-Rudiger and H. Wolfgang (eds.), *Research on Psychotherapeutic Approaches: Proceedings of the 1st European Conference on Psychotherapy Research, Trier, 1981*, Vol. 11, pp. 105–15. Frankfurt: Verlag Peter Lang.

BOZARTH, J. D. (1987), 'Further thoughts about person-centeredness', paper presented at a person-centred workshop, Warm Springs, Georgia.

CARKHUFF, R. R. (1969), *Helping and Human Relations*, Vol. 1. New York: Holt, Rinehart and Winston.

CARKHUFF, R. F. (1981), Taped interview, University of Georgia.

CARTWRIGHT, D. (1957), 'Annotated bibliography research and

NOT NECESSARILY NECESSARY BUT ALWAYS SUFFICIENT

theory construction in client-centred therapy', *Journal of Consulting Psychology*, 4, 82.

CHORDOROFF, B. (1954), 'Self-perception, perceptual defense and adjustment', *Journal of Abnormal Psychology*, 49, 508.

EGAN, G. (1982), *The Skilled Helper* (2nd ed.). Monterey, Calif.: Brooks/Cole.

ELLIS, A. (1959), 'Requisite conditions for basic personality change', *Journal of Consulting Psychology*, 23, 6.

GELSO, C. J., and CARTER, J. A. (1985), 'The relationship in counseling and psychotherapy: components, consequences, and theoretical antecedents', *The Counseling Psychologist*, 13, 159–234.

GENDLIN, G. T. (1981), Taped interview, LaJolla Program.

GORDON, T. (1970), *T.E.T.: teacher effectiveness training*. New York: New American Library.

GORDON, T. (1976), *T.E.T. in action*. New York: Wyden.

GURMAN, A. S. (1977), 'The patient's perception of the therapeutic relationship', in S. L. Garfield and A. E. Bergin (eds.), *Handbook of Psychotherapy and Behavior Change: an empirical analysis* (2nd ed.). New York: John Wiley and Sons.

KRUMBOLTZ, Z. D. (1967), 'Changing the behavior of behavior changers', *Counselor Education and Supervision*, Spring, Special Publication, 222–27.

MITCHELL, K. M., BOZARTH, J. D., and KRAUFT, C. C. (1977), 'A reappraisal of the therapeutic effectiveness of accurate empathy, non-possessive warmth, and genuineness', in A. S. Gurman and A. M. Razin (eds.), *Effective Psychotherapy: a handbook of research*. New York: Pergamon Press.

ORLINSKY, D. E., and HOWARD, K. J. (1987), 'Process and outcome in psychotherapy', in S. L. Garfield and A. E. Bergin (eds.), *Handbook of Psychotherapy and Behavioral Change: an empirical analysis*, pp. 311–81. New York: John Wiley and Sons.

PARLOFF, M. B., WASKOW, I. E., and WOLFE, B. E. (1978), 'Research on therapist variables in relation to process and outcome', in S. L. Garfield and A. E. Bergin (eds.), *Handbook of Psychotherapy and Behavior Change: an empirical analysis* (2nd ed.). New York: John Wiley and Sons.

PATTERSON, C. H. (1969), 'Necessary and sufficient conditions for psychotherapy', *The Counseling Psychologist*, 1, 2, 8–26.

PATTERSON, C. H. (1984), 'Empathy, warmth, and genuineness in psychotherapy: a review of reviews', *Psychotherapy*, 21, 431–38.

PATTERSON, C. H. (1985), *The Therapeutic Relationship: foundations for an eclectic psychotherapy*. Monterey, Ca.: Brooks/Cole.

ROGERS, C. R. (1957), 'The necessary and sufficient conditions of therapeutic personality change', *Journal of Consulting Psychology*, 21, 95–103.

ROGERS, C. R. (1959), 'A theory of therapy, personality, and interpersonal relationships, as developed in the client-centered framework', in S. Koch (ed.), *Psychology: a study of science, Vol. 3: Formulation of the person and the social context*. New York: McGraw-Hill.

ROGERS, C. R. (1961), *On Becoming a Person: a therapist's view of psychotherapy*. Boston: Houghton Mifflin.

ROGERS, C. R. (1980), *A Way of Being*. Boston: Houghton Mifflin.

ROGERS, C. R., and DIAMOND, R. F. (eds.) (1954), *Psychotherapy and Personality Change*. Chicago: University of Chicago Press.

ROGERS, C. R., GENDLIN, G. T., KEISLER, D. V., and TRAUX, C. B. (1967). *The Therapeutic Relationship and its Impact: a study of psychotherapy with schizophrenics*. Madison: University of Wisconsin Press.

SEEMAN, J. (1987), 'Round-table discussion: What areas of person-centered therapy or practice require further research? Identify specific questions on hypotheses for investigation', *Person-Centered Review*, 2, 2, 252–55.

SEEMAN, J., and RASKIN, N. J. (1953), 'Research perspectives in client-centered therapy', in O. H. Mowrer (ed.), *Psychotherapy: therapy and research*. New York: Ronald Press.

SHLIEN, J. M., and ZIMRING, F. M. (1970), 'Research directives and methods in client-centered therapy', in J. Hart and T. M. Tomlinson (eds.), *New Directions in Client-Centered Therapy*. Boston: Houghton Mifflin.

TAUSCH, R. (1978), 'Facilitative dimensions in interpersonal relations: verifying the theoretical assumptions of Carl Rogers in school, family, education, client-centered therapy, and encounter groups', *College Student Journal*, 12, 2–11.

TAUSCH, R. (1982), 'Megavitamins', in R. Ballentine (ed.), *Diet and Nutrition*, pp. 509–25. Honesdale, Pa.: Himilayan International.

TAUSCH, R. (1987a), 'Reappraisal and changing of emotions towards death and dying through imagination and person-centered group communication.' Unpublished paper.

TAUSCH, R. (1987b), 'The connection of emotions with cognitions-consequences for theoretical clarification of person-centered psy-chotherapists.' Unpublished paper.

TRUAX, C. B., and CARKHUFF, R. R. (1967), *Toward Effective Counseling and Psychotherapy: training and practice.* Chicago: Aldine.

TRUAX, C. B., and MITCHELL, K. K. (1971), 'Research on certain interpersonal skills in relation to process and outcome', in A. E. Bergin and S. L. Garfield (eds.), *Handbook of Psychotherapy and Behavior Change: an empirical analysis.* New York: John Wiley and Sons.

WATSON, N. (1984), 'The empirical status of Rogers' hypothesis of the necessary and sufficient conditions of effective therapy', in R. Levant and J. Shlien (eds.), *Client-Centered Therapy and the Person-Centered Approach: new directions in therapy, research, and practice.* New York: Prager.

# Part 2

*Creativity in Practice*

# · 5 ·

# Person-Centred Expressive Therapy: An Outcome Study

## CHARLES MERRILL AND SVEND ANDERSEN

### INTRODUCTION

Natalie Rogers* has developed a training programme called Person-Centred Expressive Therapy. It is a two-year programme consisting of four levels and offers international training for professionals who want to include expressive arts in their therapeutic and/or educational work. Passing all four levels means that participants can become certified as an Expressive Therapist. Participants may also use the workshops for personal growth. It is the intensive involvement with the learning process which has an integrative healing effect.

Expressive therapy uses expressive and creative arts in a supportive setting to facilitate growth and healing. The programme combines visual art, movement, dance, music, sound, drama, writing, guided imagery and meditation. It is a special feature of her approach that N. Rogers (N. Rogers, 1985b) combines different expressive modes and sees a connection between them which she calls the 'Creative Connection'.

Commonly, expressive therapy is separated into courses such as art therapy, dance therapy, music therapy, and creative writing. N. Rogers' idea is that the different expressive modes can mutually

* Natalie Rogers is the founder and senior faculty member of The Person-Centered Expressive Therapy Institute, P.O. Box 6528, Santa Rosa, CA 95406, USA.

nurture and enrich one another. For example, one can dramatize, sing, drum or dance a drawing, painting, or poem.

In fact, the whole training programme, as well as the daily schedule, is structured according to the idea of the Creative Connection. It alternates between meditation, art expression, reflection, conceptualization and theory, plus time for assimilation. The training is an integrative process of mind, body, emotions and spirit. Participants may develop both experiential and theoretical understanding of the healing power of expressive arts therapies and they may discover applications of the expressive arts that may be used personally and professionally.

## THE PHILOSOPHY IN PERSON-CENTRED EXPRESSIVE THERAPY

### PERSON-CENTRED THERAPY

A closer look into the single terms in the title shows that the philosophy of Carl Rogers is integrated with the expressive art modes. The term 'person-centred' is used in the way C. Rogers established the central value, placing the person at the centre of his or her own learning. The person leads the way. Qualities such as empathy, openness, acceptance, honesty and congruence are emphasized.

The programme is based on trust in the inherent impulse towards growth in every individual and group. The emphasis is on the participants' growth process, and there is confidence in the belief that every person has within an innate desire, will and know-how to strive towards self-fulfilment 'if the way is open to do so' (C. Rogers, 1969). Natalie Rogers used the metaphor, if 'the soil is fertile and the seed planted, I watch myself slowly grow and come to full blossom' (N. Rogers, 1985). The process of becoming includes the whole person and the participant is fully involved as genuine learning occurs. This learning is the basis of significant personal change in an individual.

EXPRESSIVE THERAPY

The term 'expressive art' refers to the process of creative expression with the intention of making one visible to oneself and others. Expressing oneself creatively is a growth process in and of itself. It might cause pain in experiencing fear of being known to oneself and to others, but is, at the same time, the path that may lead to self-discovery and personal growth.

By combining the different expressive modes, a process may evolve for releasing the creative potential within the individual. The participants will become familiar with different ways of expressing themselves without words, using the process of experiencing the art as a means to make known an awareness of oneself. N. Rogers helps the participants to learn a vocabulary with which they can speak through their art. She also guides them through experiences in art, fantasy and writing, which enable them to explore their inner world. N. Rogers states:

> Writing clarifies our thinking, painting changes our feelings, movement integrates our body/mind/spirit, sound opens energy channels. This is the Creative Connection as I experience it (N. Rogers, 1985b).

By learning to become more accurately aware of one's perceptions, feelings and thoughts as they are occurring, one can become more fully present in one's life. N. Rogers expresses as follows:

> This inward journey is an integrative healing process which results in the self-empowerment and a new state of consciousness of the self and the world (N. Rogers, 1988).

The expressive process is usually best experienced with a sense of openness and spontaneity. Sometimes one stays consciously aware of how the experience is affecting one, for example, how a specific movement feels or what emotions arise as one makes a certain sound on an instrument or with one's voice. Being spontaneously open to what one is about to experience is a central concept.

## EXISTENTIAL LEARNING

When people create art, it is always an aspect of the self coming into the world in the shape of a clay figure, a drawing, a rhythm, a dance, or some other mode. Creating through visual art is a very individual and personal experience which can be a very moving and powerful means for each of us to express and explore our own uniqueness. Through this process the workshop provides the individual with opportunities to pursue his or her innate desire and ability to grow and learn.

The aim is to provide the individual with opportunities to experience genuine learning and to become involved in the process of personal growth. To learn how to learn by oneself and for oneself is essential.

Genuine learning is a continuous process rather than a final end product. It is not simply the accumulation of static knowledge. Genuine learning is generated from inside the learner, not from outside sources. Only then is true meaning discovered and retained. In the workshop, genuine learning occurs as the person is directed to immediate contact with the core of his or her own aliveness, and is in real contact with the relevant problems and issues which he or she wishes to resolve.

Since genuine learning in the workshop is an affective learning process, it is experienced as moving back and forth between feelings and abstract notions. It includes the intellectual capacity for analysis and conceptualization. Insight, intellectual understanding and conceptualizing may also continue after the workshop has come to an end.

## PROCESS AND PRODUCT

Experiencing through art expression and becoming involved in the process of creatively expressing oneself seem to be the heart of the expressive art process. The focus is not on what is produced, but rather on what is experienced.

Although the participant may make attempts to understand dance, sculpture, painting, music, and writing, it is the intensive involvement with the process which provides integrative healing. The product of the creative process is the external expression of internal feelings, attitudes, perceptions, and moods. The product is what makes part of the internal self visible to oneself and to others.

When the art activity comes to a close, it is helpful to take time to assimilate and reflect upon the experience. This reflective process is often what leads to new insights and self-discoveries, especially if one views the art product with acceptance instead of with one's critical eye for 'correct' artistic style or technique.

## HOW TO OPEN THE WAY

How can a learning situation be created in which the person experiences 'congruence, unconditional positive regard, empathic understanding and acceptance' of him or herself as the genuine person he or she is (C. Rogers, 1967, p. 218)? A learning climate is provided where the person feels safe and has the courage to express him or herself through expressive art modes. The situation encourages the learner to experience as a subject rather than an object. Creating such a learning setting might be a gradual process involving both the facilitator and the participant.

Since the expressive art is a healing process in itself, one only needs a facilitator to create a safe, empathic, and stimulating environment for self-exploration through expression (N. Rogers, 1988). People only need to be encouraged to express themselves through movement, visual arts, drama, sound, and writing.

C. Rogers (1967, p. 353) mentions three inner conditions to be present in the person for the creative act. Those conditions cannot be forced, but must be permitted to emerge. First, he mentions that the person should be open to his or her experience without defensive distortion. Secondly, and perhaps this is the most fundamental condition of creativity, the source or locus of evaluative judgement is internal. Thirdly, Rogers mentions the ability to 'toy' with elements and concepts.

Those were inner psychological conditions for growth, but it is essential to look also into the psychological environmental conditions. What factors in the external environment nurture creativity? C. Rogers' (1967) experience is that psychological safety and freedom will maximize the emergence of constructive creativity.

Referring to psychological safety, C. Rogers (1967) discusses four conditions fostering constructive creativity. First of all, he mentions the acceptance of the individual as having unconditional worth. He, again, refers to the absence of external evaluation with a climate of sensitive and empathic understanding. Finally, he focuses on psychological freedom. Creativity is fostered only when the facilitator permits the individual complete freedom to express all feelings in symbolic form.

Besides psychological safety and freedom, N. Rogers (1985b) focuses on the relationship between the facilitator and the participant. She raises the question of how to provide a relationship which the person may use for his or her personal growth. How can a facilitator encourage participants to express their inner essence of truth, and guide them through experiences in art, fantasy and writing in a way which enables further self-exploration?

No method or technique will create a safe environment if the qualities of the facilitator are authoritarian, judgemental, uninterested, or interpretive. It is more a question of the philosophical frame of reference of the facilitator. N. Rogers (1985b) speaks about a deep philosophy of belief in the worth, dignity and capacity for self-direction of the person as foundation. The participant leads the way and the facilitator follows and enters the person's frame of reference in a responsive and person-centred way.

114

## THE PHYSICAL SPACE

To the extent that the workshop setting matches those inner and external psychological conditions, so will the participant exhibit creative potential. N. Rogers (1985b) has provided a physical setting that supports the psychological conditions mentioned above. The physical environment is extraordinarily exciting. Located on ten acres of land is a retreat centre with an Egyptian flavour named Isis Oasis. One can live in a retreat house, a wine barrel room or an ordinary house. A tepee, a pyramid house, a little zoo, pool, sauna, and hot tub are also provided. A dining pavilion opens out on to a vast lawn.

The group mainly works in a big old unfurnished theatre with a stage and balcony. The daily schedule is tight and here is an example of a typical day.

```
 7.30–  8.15 Movement and meditation (Session I)
 8.30–  9.15 Breakfast
 9.30–12.15 Session II
12.30–  1.15 Lunch
 1.30–  3.00 Rest and assimilation
 3.00–  4.15 Session III
 4.30–  5.45 Session IV
 6.00–  6.45 Dinner
 6.45–  7.30 Free time
 7.30–  9.30 Session V
```

All kinds of activities such as dancing, writing, singing, conversation, drawing, painting, making videos, counselling, theory lectures, playing rhythm instruments, art performance, working with clay, and being together are encouraged. Within two days all the walls are covered with participants' drawings and paintings. Soon afterwards, one will find sculptures as well. Participants work individually, in pairs, small groups and in the group as a whole. All kinds of art material are available and the participants are encouraged to use them freely for self-expression.

## PARTICIPANT FOLLOW-UP STUDY

We, as researchers, found it important to give voice to the participants who had attended the programme during the six years since it began in 1985. They were asked to tell the researchers, in their own words, about their experience in the person-centred expressive therapy training. The plan of the study was to invite participants to report how the workshop(s) had affected their personal growth. The focus was not on the training programme in its four levels or on an evaluation of the training aspects. The participants were involved on different levels and with different purposes. They may have participated with the goal of becoming a professional in expressive therapy or to achieve personal growth in its own right.

We were interested in learning if participants had made a perceptual shift or change regarding themselves and the people around them. Since we were concerned about deep emotional learning, it was difficult for some participants to find verbal expression for their experience of growth. It was also difficult when it came to writing down their experiences and feelings, and describing the tone and atmosphere of the workshop setting.

The intellectual part is secondary, although it is in the light of conscious reality that things have to be seen, understood and integrated and lived. The researchers thought that the participants might be able to reflect on their expressive therapy experience and on how the workshop(s) had given meaning to their inner dialogue and to their attitudes and behaviour. What was the effect of an intensive experience where one was exposed to different modes of learning in an atmosphere of expectation and acceptance?

## DESCRIPTION OF PARTICIPANTS IN STUDY

Participants in the Person-Centered Therapy Institute comprised counsellors, educators, and graduate students from all around the United States, Europe and several South American and Asian countries. The work of Natalie Rogers has an international reputation, and so there was a very interesting mix of participants in the training workshops. One of the reasons we were interested in conducting this study was the unusual and varied backgrounds of the individuals in the training.

The respondents' ages ranged from twenty-two to sixty-six; twenty (66 per cent) were between thirty-six and fifty.

## METHODS USED

Open-ended questionnaires asked former participants to describe a situation in one of their workshops that stood out as especially meaningful to them. They were asked to reflect on how the situation about which they wrote was meaningful to them. We wanted to know if remembered workshop situations encouraged former participants to have an inner dialogue with themselves. What we meant by inner dialogue was the possibility that what happened for participants might have given new meaning to their lives. We were also interested in knowing if participants' behaviour and actions changed as a result of their workshop experience.

A second open-ended question asked respondents to reflect on how their 'way-of-being' might be at least partially related to their personal learnings. With such a question, we were hoping for an indication of deeper-level personal change. One additional question asked respondents to give feedback about how writing down their expressive therapy experiences made them feel. The thirty-two former participants who responded to the mailed questionnaire formed a large enough group to give a reliable range of significant expressive arts workshop situations.

## LIMITATIONS OF THE STUDY

The mailing list consisted of two hundred former participants, and the responses received were thirty-two completed questionnaires from individuals who had completed at least Level I of the training.

No attempt was made to evaluate the responses based on levels. It was our opinion that a significant event might happen at any of the four levels, and it was the meaning of that particular situation which we were hopeful of obtaining. Level I was six days in length and many participants continued in Level II, which was an additional week.

Respondents had completed Level I between 1985 (which was when the Person-Centered Expressive Therapy Institute began formal training) and 1990. Respondents who participated in the training more recently may have been affected by the 'halo' effect more than respondents who participated in earlier years.

Evaluation of the written responses was impressionistic and we limited our analysis to searching for the inherent structure imbedded in each co-participant's response. Therefore, our results are tentative and based on thematic content analysis, following the phenomenological research method of Amedeo Giorgi summarized by Donald Polkinghorne (1989).

We have the participants' reported statements about significant situations which affected them and we have attempted to be careful not to read more into the responses. A limitation of this approach is that we are dealing with respondents' memories about specific situations that may have happened several years in the past. At best we hope we have been able to cluster the significant themes referred to by the respondents.

## RESULTS AND DISCUSSION

As we understand the written responses, it is evident that our findings are thematic and impressionistic. We have drawn from the meaning units in a way that is psychological but which stays close to what we think the respondents meant. We began by reviewing the activities participants emphasized in their written responses. Of the thirty-two respondents, exactly one half (sixteen) wrote about their creation of a significant drawing, painting, sculpture or collage. An example was given by one respondent who approached a drawing from a process perspective:

> When we were directed to translate our feelings into some art form I stormed outside and started making a big angry painting. As I worked on it I felt sort of detached and began watching myself acting on my anger to create something. It was almost like the painting was creating me. (Respondent 17)

This excerpt suggests that a participant may express some unexplored aspect of him or herself through the art form without using words. Participants came to trust other modes of expression and exploration of feelings, images and possibilities. There was a valuing of whatever form a participant chose to use as long as it did not impinge upon another. The above-cited response to anger was expressed through the drawing and represented a different relationship to this often suppressed emotion.

The next most frequent activity involved various forms of movement including dancing alone and/or with others to music, acting out a drawing, or moving to a poem being read aloud. Seven of the respondents reflected upon some form of personal experience with movement. A powerful example of how dance can touch one at some depth is given in the following example:

> I danced what for me was my emotional life story to that point. It was a painful dance and one that drew me down, down, down, into profound feeling. I dared myself . . . to feel the truth in its time and intensity. It was the riskiest work I have ever done. (Respondent 3)

The beauty of person-centred work, as offered through expressive therapy modes, is that the person is central and can freely choose what will be used as self-exploration tools whether it be drawing, painting, movement or some other modality.

The next most frequently mentioned activity was writing. Approaches to writing included free writing, poetry, stories, and journal-writing. Six of the thirty-two respondents referred to one of these as personally meaningful and improving their inner sense of themselves. Here is a rich example of how writing affected one respondent's life:

> We were . . . writing about a spirit guide we had met in an earlier meditation. [After writing about her spirit guide] . . . They conducted a ceremony for me in which the lesson was 'even darkness can be welcomed because I always have myself'. This experience empowered me to take the center of my own life in a unique way. (Respondent 10)

Sometimes the experience of writing was felt as complete in itself, and at other times participants combined writing with another activity such as movement or some dramatic enactment, as the above example illustrates.

Six respondents wrote about a dramatic event such as role playing, improvisation, gestures, masks, mime, or some form of guided imagery as helping them connect with an inner wisdom. An unusual example by an older participant follows.

> When Natalie led us in the drama of The Village, I became the wise old woman. Others came to me for comfort and closeness. I liked this role; I think the process helped me accept the fact of my ageing. I began to see myself as one who has garnered a lot of wisdom which might be shared. (Respondent 14)

Two other respondents wrote about how music and making sounds on a rhythm and percussion instrument were significant, and one person remembered meditation as important. Here is an example of how sound and rhythm affected one person.

> Playing the musical instruments, particularly the percussion ones, and creating rhythms that fed upon each other, was energizing and satisfying. It strengthened my belief in spontaneity and risk taking, that I could try the unfamiliar and create something with myself and others. (Respondent 7)

It appears from the responses that choosing to participate in some form of creative activity helped respondents feel better about themselves. It seems that the process of creating something, participating with others in a group or working on some solitary project gave inspiration and encouragement to individuals to express themselves more openly and with less fear of being judged.

The expressive therapy training workshops provided participants with a wide range of experiential learning activities, and each person was encouraged to find his or her own areas of exploration and expression. We emphasize the exploration aspect. Judgements were not made on the participants' artistic abilities or products, but instead, each individual was encouraged to allow the creative process to affect him or her in whatever way felt congruent with the chosen media.

## SIGNIFICANT LEARNINGS

Carl Rogers (1967) spoke many times about significant learning for the person. He specifically stated:

> . . . significant learning is more than accumulation of facts. It is learning which makes a difference in the individual's behavior, in the course of action he chooses in the future, in his attitude and in his personality (1967, pp. 167–75).

Rogers' view of significant learning seems an appropriate one as we have sorted the meaning units into psychological language. He also spells out more closely the various aspects of significant learning. The person more fully accepts him or herself and his or her feelings. He or she feels more self-confident and self-directing. When we analysed the responses on this dimension we found that seventeen respondents referred in some way to feeling more self-accepting. An example from one respondent follows:

> I am a different person than I might have been . . . This work encouraged me to believe in myself! It gave me the courage to

start my own business. It gave me tools to fight the fears that were holding me back. (Respondent 2)

Another related dimension is that the person comes to see him or herself differently. Nine respondents indicated that they felt and saw themselves in a new way. One person put it this way:

When I returned home I felt really transformed. I felt much more . . . grounded in this world, more sexual. My voice was deeper. I felt my center lower in my body, around my solar plexus. I was greatly empowered . . . (Respondent 1)

Yet another of C. Rogers' significant learning dimensions concerns adopting more realistic goals for oneself. Five respondents referred to being more realistic about their goals and plans for their lives as a result of the expressive therapy training. One respondent expressed it this way:

I am more willing to spend time with myself, getting to know myself better. I also am a bit more careful about choosing actions until I have some sense of where these motivations arise from. (Respondent 12)

As mentioned earlier, respondents reported more self-acceptance. Interestingly, six also reported that they were more accepting of others. It seems that when a person is willing to value him or herself in a non-judgemental way, others are valued for the way they are rather than how one expects them to be. A telling example of accepting another follows:

My personal life is different now, I have learned to relate to others, including my children, in a more realistic way, which of course helps me to have less expectations towards me and others, and therefore, judge less and accept more of what comes . . . (Respondent 30)

## THE CREATIVE CONNECTION AND PERSONAL GROWTH

Personal development has been written about by many humanistic writers including Natalie Rogers herself. In her book *Emerging Woman* (1980), she discloses her own unique journey towards greater autonomy and personhood. Her inner journey towards emancipation from the oppressiveness of society's expectations about being a dutiful wife and mother has been a model for many women. In other words, N. Rogers is a pioneer in women's liberation as well as an innovator of a perspective on person-centred learning.

Her explorations on the Creative Connection (1985b) have been demonstrated through her expressive therapy training workshops. N. Rogers describes the Creative Connection as:

> . . . the connection between movement, art, writing and sound. When we move with awareness it opens us to profound feelings which can then be expressed in color, line or form. When we write immediately after movement or art work there is a free flow from the unconscious . . . (1985a)

The Creative Connection involves personal growth as a central tenet of the creative process and ties in theoretically with C. Rogers' significant learning dimensions discussed earlier. In sorting out the specific factors we think are related to the Creative Connection and personal growth, we see several exemplified by many of the respondents in this study.

Although impressionistic, the analysis of written responses showed all thirty-two referring to a process of *integrative healing* resulting from their expressive therapy work. The experience of feeling more integrated with one's inner self was mentioned many times. Below is an example that summarizes the over-arching integrative aspect of the Creative Connection:

> I recall a process in which the group was led in a guided visualization. We went within and found a door behind which were our sub-personalities. We opened the door and let them out,

encountering several and asking each who they were, what they have to give us, and what they wanted. This process was very *integrating* for me . . . helping me to acknowledge, hear and love these parts of myself . . . (Respondent 9)

Another dimension we found was that almost one half (fourteen) of the respondents reported feeling self-empowered as essential to their personal growth. This aspect is similar to developing greater self-confidence and self-acceptance discussed earlier as part of significant learning. One participant expressed how she felt based on expressive therapy training:

As a result of these workshops, I am much more interested in finding *my own expression and honoring it.* I respect my uniqueness, even when that uniqueness is so different from anything encouraged by the culture I live in. (Respondent 11)

The data revealed another aspect of the Creative Connection to be a new consciousness about not only one's inner self but the world of relationships at work and in the larger community. Twelve respondents reported that their consciousness of themselves and others had shifted internally as a result of their expressive therapy experiences. Below is given a very poignant example of a shift in consciousness.

As a result of a one-day workshop I got an inner image, and experience of the part of me that is unaffected by life, the part of me *complete in its 'being'.* It greatly reduced my fear when I felt it. (Respondent 6)

We also want to mention that six respondents changed their jobs or careers and nine felt that their professional skills were enhanced by their expressive therapy training. One respondent put it this way:

The training opened me to the path to become a facilitator using art and movement. I learned when we express things truly in us, we can make deep connection with ourselves . . . I think it helped me to become a more effective facilitator. I just taught a series of ten classes of expressive therapy and I loved to look at people's work and process. (Respondent 15)

Others indicated that they were able to discover some new aspect of themselves and to creatively solve some inner conflict with their new expressive modes.

## CRITICAL FEEDBACK

A few respondents reported mixed feelings about their expressive therapy work. One person was bothered by some ethically question-able actions by the institute staff. The respondent's own words are as follows:

. . . in a general way, feel I have benefitted from the experience. I also had one unpleasant experience at the end of the workshop. However, it did color my overall impression of the professional-ism and ethics of the staff. (Respondent 7)

Another respondent gave a less than enthusiastic response to her workshop experience. She learned more about herself from the training, but was already well versed in personal growth modes. She expresses it this way:

. . . it is impossible for me to attribute a great 'AHA' to the workshop. The workshop certainly reinforced how important it is to allow time and space to simply 'be'. (Respondent 5)

There were very few statements that were not enthusiastic, but almost all the thirty-two respondents felt some significant inner change happened. Of course we do not know what the former participants who did not respond to the questionnaire might have said. Perhaps some did not answer because they did have mixed reactions. Some people do not like open-ended essay-type questions. On the whole, those who participated in this study did find something meaningful in the training workshop.

## SUMMARY AND CONCLUSIONS

In a non-statistical study such as this one, our data was impressionistic and thematic. The questionnaire was open-ended to allow for the fullest possible response. Each individual had a unique experience with expressive therapy modes emphasizing different areas of the training. Some participants preferred drawing over movement or group participation. Some liked more dramatic and/or musical activities. Dance was yet another mode that many respondents reported as meaningful.

The data does indicate that all participants experienced some form of integrative healing and greater self-awareness. Many reported inner changes as a result of their workshop experience. The accepting climate and non-intrusive facilitation helped participants feel safe and yet challenged to explore their feelings and established ways of being. The group experience was central to most participants because they felt supported and encouraged to share their artistic and creative work with other participants.

As mentioned earlier, the creative process was valued, not the artistic value of the product. The beauty of N. Rogers' work is that she so skilfully educated her staff to provide conditions that were enhancing of one's inner expression of feeling and thought. Expectations were minimal, yet participants were expected to take responsibility for their actions and to respect other participants' right to do their own personal work.

The most reported learnings ranged from developing greater self-confidence to feeling less fearful and more willing to take risks. Discovering some new inner strength, finding the courage to create and to share their process and/or product with the larger group were reported by almost all respondents.

126

Although many participants reported that they felt empowered to change some external situation in their lives, the primary goal of the expressive therapy training seems to be to provide a learning climate that facilitates inner changes of attitude and feeling towards personal growth.

The data analysis shows that this goal is being realized by most of the former participants who responded to the questionnaire. A point that was also mentioned by many respondents is the need for continuing expressive therapy work after the workshops had ended. The institute regularly offers follow-up workshops for one day, a weekend, or a week. Several respondents were able to continue on their own with no follow-up. On the whole, the learnings seemed to be permanent for most respondents and the transferability of learning to other personal and professional situations was evident in many of the responses.

In closing, we find that there is a need for an additional follow-up study that includes in-depth personal interviews with former participants. However, based on the results of the data, our conclusion is that the expressive therapy methods offered through the Person-Centered Expressive Therapy Institute are a major step forward in furthering person-centred learning.

REFERENCES

KNANNA, M. (1989), 'A phenomenological investigation of creativity in person-centered expressive therapy.' Unpublished doctoral dissertation. University of Tennessee, Knoxville.

POLKINGHORNE, D. E. (1989), 'Phenomenological research methods', in R. S. Valle and Steen Halling (eds.), *Existential-Phenomenological Perspectives in Psychology*. New York: Plenum Press.

ROGERS, C. R. (1967), *On Becoming a Person*. London: Constable.

ROGERS, C. R. (1969), *Freedom to Learn*. Columbus, Ohio: Charles E. Merrill.

ROGERS, N. (1988), 'Theory notes'. Unpublished. Person-Centered Expressive Therapy Institute, Santa Rosa, California.

ROGERS, N. (1985a), *Express Yourself*. Association of Humanistic Psychology, Perspective, April.

ROGERS, N. (1985b), *The Creative Connection: a person-centered approach to expressive therapy*. (Available from Person-Centered Expressive Therapy Institute, 1515 Riebli Rd., Santa Rosa, California 95404.)

ROGERS, N. (1980), *Emerging Woman: a decade of midlife transition*. Point Reyes, California: Personal Press. (Available from Person-Centered Expressive Therapy Institute, 1515 Riebli Rd., Santa Rosa, California 95404.)

· 6 ·

# Creating a Workable Distance to Overwhelming Images: Comments on a Session Transcript

## MIA LEIJSSEN

### INTRODUCTION

The following is a transcript of part of an experiential therapy session, together with my subsequent reflections upon the work as it develops. This session came about after I had been called in by a less experienced therapist to help the client* who was overwhelmed by terrifying images. Focusing helped the client to put the images at a distance and then to watch them as a means to open underlying feelings.

Focusing is paying attention inwardly to the unclear sense of something 'there'. This process may arise spontaneously in the client or it may need facilitation. The way to touch the inside felt sense can be taught. The teaching of focusing is usually presented as a six-step process: 1. clearing a space; 2. attending to a felt sense; 3. finding a handle; 4. resonating; 5. asking; 6. receiving. (Gendlin, 1981.)

However during therapy, it is not recommended to 'teach' focusing; here it is preferable that the therapist models the more general focusing attitude of waiting in the presence of the not yet speakable and being receptive to the not yet formed. The 'steps' can be referred to as 'subtasks' or 'micro-processes' offered at certain

---

* I wish to thank Angela (client's pseudonym) for her 'share' in this chapter. The transcript is an unchanged version of part of the session. Therapist and client are female; hence the personal pronoun 'she' is used.

moments in psychotherapy. (See in this respect Leijssen, 1990.)

To illustrate the integration of focusing in psychotherapy, the transcript of a part of this experiential therapy session will be alternated by descriptions of the micro-processes client and therapist are going through and attention will be given to the focusing attitude and specific interventions of the therapist to facilitate the client's process.

## TRANSCRIPT AND COMMENTS*

C1: Do you actually want me to tell you what it was like?
T1: Wait, let's just start with where you are now.
C2: Hm ... (sighs) ... actually the same, very distraught (weeps, sobs) ... very scared.

The client is in an overwhelmed state, she is too close with what's there (A. Weiser, 1991). This is a clue to begin to offer the micro-process of 'clearing a space'. The crux of this micro-process concerns making a friendly accepting space where the client can be with a sense of separatedness and where she can feel that she is OK. When the therapist accompanies the client in the creation of a workable distance from an unbearable or overwhelming problem, there is a whole set of 'finding distance' moves. However it is very important that the client can receive empathic responses from the therapist and process suggestions that are tailored exactly to the specific problem at that moment.

T2: Very scared. Do you feel more comfortable when I'm close to you?
C3: Yes.
T3: OK, then I come closer (T edges up to C and puts her hand on C's knee).

* In commenting on the transcript, the model of Rice, Greenberg and Elliott (in press) was of particular help.

The therapist making physical contact with the client during a therapy session is very unusual. Here the therapist chooses to do so because the client doesn't make any eye contact and is so overwhelmed by her fear that she hardly seems to notice the presence of the therapist. The therapist offers the physical holding as a way of 'containing' the client in trouble.

C4: (sobs and sighs) The feelings come and go in waves (sighs). It's a very scary feeling and then . . . a sort of peace, like now. (T: Hm.)
(15 second silence) I feel as if I'm on the edge of something. (T: Hm.)
(22 second silence) I'm just feeling the peace now.

The client experiences some relief, which indicates she has found some distance. Client and therapist adopt the focusing attitude by quietly remaining present with the not yet speakable.

T4: Now you are in the peace of it.
C5: Right.
T5: There is a peaceful part in it and a scareful part in it, yes.
C6: It's a sort of drifting. (T: Hm.) Sort of sucking down; a kind of going down and sucking down. (T: Hm.)
(25 second silence) (sobs)
Like . . . (inarticulate) skating down. (sobs) (T gives handkerchief to C.) I'm just lying there for the moment. Just, just lying there. (T: Hm.)
T6: So, there is a piece in it where you feel peaceful, but then in another part you feel scary.

The therapist evokes the scary part, because she feels this peaceful part is not the result of something that has been resolved, but rather a temporary state of relief due to the 'containment' of the therapist. The client isn't yet at a productive 'working distance' between self and problem.

C7: Right, yes (frightened). And I'm getting the eye again. (sobs, hyperventilates)

The client is completely overwhelmed by an image with a hallucinatory quality and she loses contact with reality and with the therapist.

T7: Yes, listen to me, listen to me, listen to me, please open your eyes. Look to me, yes. Listen, this scary part . . . follow me . . . (C: Yes.) This scary part, that's not you. (C: Right.) You are Angela. (C: Yes.) . . . OK, you stay Angela. (C: Right.) OK?

The therapist tries to restore reality contact by 'calling the client back' in the contact with the therapist, by disidentifying her from the scary part and by reminding her of her name.

C8: Yes.
T8: The scary part that's here.

The therapist gives the scary part a place at some distance from the client in order to make the disidentification very concrete. Client and therapist are working at the subtask of finding a productive 'working distance' between the client and the problem.

C9: Right.
T9: Here.
C10: Yes.
T10: That's not you, and we can even put it farther away. (C hyperventilates.) OK. You are Angela.
C11: Yes.
T11: This whole scary part (C: Yes.), we put it on a safe distance.
C12: Right.
T12: We together, we are trying to make a safe distance.
C13: Right . . . yeah. (hyperventilating diminishes)
T13: Let's first find out together, how we can make a safe distance.

132

C14: Right.

T14: A distance that feels good for you.

C15: OK . . . Right.
(16 second silence) (sobs, takes a deep breath, sighs heavily)

T15: So first, the first thing we are going to do now is making this safe distance.

C16: Right.

T16: A distance that you feel safe. Yes?

C17: Yes.

T17: How . . . how can we do it in a way that you feel safe? Can we . . . put it in another place where you have your hand on the door and the door is closed and you can open or close it, or, is there another image you feel we can work with . . . to put in that scary thing. Look for your image.

The use of metaphors is a way to find a comfortable relationship with overwhelming experiences. The therapist guides this process, but she tries to engage the client in finding the metaphor that fits with her experience.

C18: Right. (calms down)

T18: And if there is one, tell me about it.

C19: Well I feel that hum, what's happening is a sort of . . . a kind of invasion (T: Hm.) like a seeping sow (sighs heavily).

T19: Wait a moment, wait a moment. First we, we look how you can stay at a safe distance (C: Right.) to the scary thing. That's what we first do.

The therapist is afraid that the client isn't making distance, therefore she repeats the task instructions.

C20: Right. I'm trying to think of ways to counteract it. And I can only think that I shout it back at the moment. (T: Hm.) Pushing away (T: Hm.), that's all, at the moment, that's all I'm feeling, it's a wanting to push it away.

Now the client is in the task of making distance and she involves the image of 'pushing away'.

T20: A wanting to push it away.
C21: Right.
T21: Yeah. Let's push it away . . .
C22: OK, fine.
T22: In a distance that feels safe for you.
C23: Right. (sobs) (10 second silence) (deep breath)
T23: So we push this away.
C24: Right. I'm trying to push, in my mind I'm focusing on pushing away.
T24: Yes. And push it far enough.
C25: Right, I'm doing it . . . I think I'm doing it . . . I'm moving it away, I think.
T25: You feel you have pushed it away?
C26: Well, not very far, but it's moving away gradually. (T: Hm.) Yeah.
T26: It needs still more?
C27: It's still quite close.
T27: Yes, it needs more distance still.
C28: I think so.
T28: Yes, OK, push it away (C: Right.), until you find the right distance for you. (C: Hm.) The distance you really feel safe with.
C29: Hm. (10 second silence) (sighs)
    It's feeling easier. (T: Hm.) All right, that's feeling easier.

The client feels more separate from the problem. This usually results in an experience of relief.

T29: You find the right distance for you?
C30: Yeah.
T30: Tell me about it, is it . . .

It's not only important that the client feels separate from the problem. A good working distance also implies that the client can stay

134

in contact with the problem. So the therapist initiates this subtask of contacting the problem at a distance.

C31: It's about ... (points at the direction)
T31: It's there ... (points at the same direction)
C32: Right, it's over there.
T32: Over there. How far? Is there something in between you and that threatening thing?

As it is not clear how much the client is in contact with reality, the therapist stays at a very concrete level and makes several contact reflections as is done in Pre-therapy (see Prouty, 1990).

C33: No, there's nothing in between.
T33: Nothing in between, only a distance ... OK.
C34: Yes, it's just distance.
T34: Just distance, yeah, it's over there.
C35: Right. (T: Hm.) Mhm, like six foot or something like that.
T35: Mhm, yeah. You feel safe with ...
C36: I'm feeling better.
T36: ... that there (C: Hm.) at that distance. (C: Right.) OK. So, you stay in this safe place (C: Right.), and that thing, that threatening thing stays over there (C: Right.), it doesn't come closer. (C: Right.) Not at all. (C: OK.) OK? (C: Mhm.) And you stay here with me.
C37: Right. OK. (6 second silence)
T37: Just take your time to ... to feel this: you being here. You Angela, being here in a safe place.

After having ensured the working distance (T36), the therapist invites the client to experience how it feels to be an 'I' without the identification with the problem. This can be a strengthening and healing experience.

C38: Mhm. (26 second silence)

The C 'receives' the changed feeling. The receiving process often takes place during silence.

T38: How does this feel . . . ?

C39: I'm letting go . . . (T: Hm.) gradually. I feel like, a kind of an unwinding.

T39: Mhm. It's important to feel this unwinding. (C: Mhm.) Yes. Mhm.

C40: Mhm. (54 second silence)

The micro-process of receiving is still continuing.

T40: How are you at the moment?

C41: Fine, I feel fine actually.

T41: Yes, OK.

C42: I'm feeling quite strong now actually. (T: Hm.) (T: OK.) It's feeling quite good. (T: Hm.) Hm.

T42: Now . . . now we both know that over there (C: Mhm.) there is still that threatening thing you are very scared of. (C: Mhm.) You stay at your safe place with me. (C: Hm.) You don't let that come in again. (C: Right.) We are just going to look together to that very scary thing over there. (C: Mhm.) But we don't let it come closer. (C: Right.) OK? We stay together in this safe place. (C: Hm.) Is that OK?

C43: Yes, that's fine. Mhm.

T43: So, if you look at what you know that is there at that distance . . . what . . . how does that whole feel towards you? What does it arise in you? (13 second silence)

After the consolidation of the good working distance (T42) and the confirmation of the client that she feels safe in allowing herself to look at the scary thing in the presence of the therapist (C43), the therapist introduces the next micro-process: 'forming a felt sense'. In this task the client is asked to place her inward-turned attention on the problem, in order to allow a holistic felt sense to form.

C44: I don't know.
T44: Take your time.
    (33 second silence)

The therapist encourages the focusing attitude of receptive waiting and allows the client to take time. The formation of a felt sense requires time and silence. This step is largely non-verbal for clients.

C45: A kind of ... hum ... , a mixture of things I think. (T: Hmh.) Something to do with darkness and something to do with, hum ... I can only ... can I give you an image?

As soon as the client tries to put her experience into words, she is in the next micro-process: 'finding a handle'. This client progresses spontaneously to this step, without any direction or prompting from the therapist. It is remarkable that an image often presents itself as the expression of the complex experience. Metaphors have the advantage of catching the essentials of the still unspeakable and expressing it in its full complexity with just a few words.

T45: Hmh. Please do.
C46: A sort of fog.
T46: A sort of fog.
C47: Mhm, a creeping fog. (T: Mhm.) That's what I'm sort of picking up. (T: Mhm.) A creeping fog.
T47: A creeping fog. (C: Hm.) That's, how it feels like ...

The most important thing for the therapist to do at this stage is to listen empathically and to reflect what the client expresses. The client is supported to develop an initial verbal label or pictural symbol for the non-verbal felt sense, by means of a kind of 'dialogue' with it. The dialogue is continued in the next step, where the emergent labels are resonated or checked against the felt sense.

In this case something very special is happening: the therapist, not being a native English speaker, doesn't understand the words 'creeping fog'. Nevertheless she decides to wait to ask for some explanation and she reflects the keywords.

C48: That's exactly what it feels like. (T:  OK.) I recognized it. (T: Mhm.) Yeah, it's creeping.

T48: Mhm, creeping.

C49: Mhm. Very low-lying. (T: Hm.) Close to the ground. (T: Hm.)
(17 second silence)

T49: That's how it feels to you. (C: Hm.) Creeping.

C50: Hm.
(35 second silence)

T50: Is that the complete feeling or are there other things around? Or . . .

C51: There were in the last session. But in this one, it's just the creeping fog at the moment.

T51: Just a creeping fog.

C52: Hm, that was there in the last session as well.

T52: Hm. I don't know what it means, 'a creeping fog'. Can you tell me something more, so I can really get the quality of the creeping fog? (C: Hm.) I don't understand this. Sorry.

The therapist feels that the client can't deepen the process with only 'technical reflection' from therapist's side. This might be an illustration of the importance of the therapist really understanding what she is reflecting.

C53: Mhm (sighs), that's all right . . . uhm. Something very intense, menacing and a kind of flimsy at the same time.

T53: Flimsy?

C54: Yeah . . . uhm . . . like a fog, you go through it, it's thin. You can move through it.

T54: What's a fog? I don't know what a fog is.

C55: A mist.

T55: Yes, OK. OK.

C56: A mist. (T: Hmh.) You can move through it. (T: Yes.) It's thick.

T56: Yes, OK, yes, I understand.

C57: And it moves very slowly. (T: Yes, hm.) And it creeps. (T: Mhm.) That's all I can say, it creeps across the ground and it moves towards me.

T57: Oh, it's like that (C: Right.) and moves very slowly (C: Yeah.) and it's thick.

C58: Yes, it is thick, yeah. And it moves through things.

T58: It moves through things. Oh yeah, yes.

Especially in this phase where the client looks for words to describe her complex feeling, it is important to be very non-directive and to retain loaded words. Indeed, if the therapist changes the client's expression, the client might loose the specific loading connected with the word.

C59: Yes, like a fog moves through things and covers them up.

T59: Hm. It's that what you felt! 'It covers me up.'

Here is an experiential shift in the therapist! Now she understands at a deeper level what's happening. The part of the reflection, done in the first person, has a vivid and evocative quality, expressing that right now the therapist is experiencing as the client.

C60: Right (T: Hm.), Yes. (T: Hm.) That's right, right, that's it (deep sigh). It was covering me up.

Being exactly understood leads to a big relief and simultaneous experiential shift in the client.

T60: Hm, yes, now I understand you.

C61: Yes (sighs). I'm getting in touch with it again.

T61: It's somehow very difficult to let it over there?

C62: Yes, it is something . . .

T62: It moves very slowly and it covers you up.

The therapist felt that T61 was somehow out of the client's track, so by repeating previous keywords of the client, the therapist tries to encourage the client to continue on her own track.

C63: Right. (T: Hm.) And there is something about me in it. (T: Hm.) But I don't know what that is yet.

After being correctly understood, the client is able to continue and unfold more elements of the felt sense.

T63: Hm. But you feel: 'There's something about me in it'?

The therapist helps the client to maintain the focusing attitude by receiving the new element without going 'prematurely' into explanations.

C64: Right.
T64: In that fog or . . .
C65: Oh, a kind of to do with this moving.
T65: With this slowly moving?
C66: Yeah. (T: Hmh.) Like it's moving around me. (T: Hmh.) And it's something about me . . . wanting it to move around me and not wanting it to move around me. A kind of beckoning and not beckoning.
T66: Yes. It's not quite sure what you really want with that?
C67: Possibly.
T67: Somehow wanting and not wanting. (C: Mhm.) Hum. (C: Hm.) So.
C68: Mhm . . . Mhm . . . I can't say anything more at the moment.
T68: Mhm. But that seems something really important that . . . it has to do something with you . . . wanting and not wanting. (C: Right.) OK. (C: Mhm.) This ambiguity. (C: Mhm.) Yes.

The therapist feels she was not quite right in T66, so in T67 she returns to previous keywords and confirms the message of the client by an empathic response in T68.

C69: Hmh. A kind of rolling as well.

The felt sense unfolds itself further in the back and forth movement between symbolization and what is felt.

T69: Rolling.
C70: Rolling towards me.
T70: What's that rolling?
C71: (sighs) Rolling down.
T71: Mhm ... I'm not quite sure that I really capture what it means for you.
C72: Well, creeping and rolling. At the same time. I can't explain it.
T72: It has to do with this slowly moving thing?
C73: Right.
T73: ... Where you feel you ... go in also, or that comes into you and ... ?
C74: It comes, it comes into me and moves up in me somehow. Like it moves up my spine.
T74: As if it seems to possess you. (C: Mhm.) Is it like that?
C75: Yes, it is.
T75: It possesses you.
C76: Yes, right (sighs).
T76: There's something that takes possession of you.
C77: Right. Mhm. (T: Mhm ... yeah.) (13 second silence) It has a connection with something white. (T: Yes?) Like fog is white.

The therapist has some difficulty with the language, but she tries very hard to understand (T71, T72, T73) and finally touches a deeper meaning of it (T74), which causes again a relief in the client and enables her to go on to a different quality of the image.

T77: Yeah, it has a colour: white.

C78: White. (T: Mhm.) It moves over darkness, but it's white.

T78: Mhm. So these are meaningful qualities in it. (C: Mhm.) Something white but it moves over darkness. (C: Mhm . . . mhm . . . hm.) Something that takes possession of you.

C79: Mm. It moves over me.

T79: It moves over you.

C80: Mm. Invades me. (T: Hmhm.) Hm.

T80: You are invaded by it.


The micro-process of checking or resonating involves an extensive back-and-forth search between a series of labels and an evolving felt sense. The therapist's most important job in this step is helping the client to maintain the contact between felt sense and potential labels until the sense of rightness or fit emerges.


C81: Right. (T: Hm.) It kind of attaches itself all the way around me. (T: Mhm.) And earlier I had this sense of . . . of me being a nucleus . . . and the thing being like the edge of a cell.

T81: Mm . . . You being a nucleus? What's a nucleus . . . precisely?

C82: It's . . . biology. (T: Yes.) A cell in the body. (T: Yes.) It's the main middle bit. (T: Hm.) Like the brain of it.

T82: Yes, I understand.

C83: And the whiteness is around.

T83: Yes, I understand.

C84: Like a cell (T: Hm.) edging.

T84: Yes. As if you are completely absorbed (C: Right.) by it (C: Yes.) . . . and at the same time you are the nucleus of it.

C85: Right. (T: Yes.) That feels very . . . that feels very . . . exact. (T: Mhm.)
(20 second silence).
And it's a sucking feeling somehow connected with that too. (T: Hm?) Being sucked.

The client feels deeply understood by T84. She can stay in the focusing attitude of waiting silently with the still unformed and receive some new elements.

T85: Being sucked?

C86: Yeah, being sucked into it. (T: Hm.) Being centre and being sucked into it. (T: Hm.) Like the darkness in the middle of the whiteness.

T86: What's sucked, being sucked precisely? Like a baby does when he takes in the milk, is that sucking?

C87: Yes, yes.

T87: You feel that you are sucked in it?

C88: Yes, like moving down. (T: Hm, yes.) (sighs) Yes.

T88: 'I feel sucked in it.' (C: Yes.) That's how you feel about it.

C89: Yes, hm.

T89: Something that is very hard to resist?

C90: Hm, hm. Yeah.
    (12 second silence)

T90: So you have this very powerful image of being the nucleus of a cell (C: Hm.) and a feeling of being sucked into something. That's a very powerful image. (C: Hm.) Can you try to feel what in your life feels like that? Do you somewhere in your ongoing life now, recognize some of those qualities that you describe with this image? Some of the same qualities . . .

The therapist introduces a new step. Until now the client has expressed several qualities of the felt sense. However a felt sense is not just 'feelings'. A felt sense is always 'about something'; a complex of feelings connected to something in one's life.

C91: I think it got something to do with . . . I don't want to intellectualize.

T91: Hm, just what's coming up?

C92: (sighs) The only thing that reminds me of that is being in relationships with people. Feeling off balance . . . sometimes.

The meaning of the felt sense begins to open.

T92: Being out of balance?

C93: Yeah. Being sucked in ... (T: Yes.) into a relationship. Feeling a bit swamped. Yes. That's the only thing I can connect to.

T93: That's OK. That seems meaningful. (C: Hm.) That being sucked into something, that's what happens with you in relationships?

The therapist resonates the emergence of the new element and the client receives it in a silence in C94 and feels ready to move further.

C94: Yeah. (T: Mhm.)
(12 second silence)
So I want to keep things at bay.

T94: Mhm. It's something that you feel you want (C: Mhm.): keeping things at bay?

The therapist resonates the handle, the client checks it against the felt sense.

C95: Hm. (7 second silence)

T95: Something as a response to this being sucked in?

C96: Yeah. (T: Mm.) Like it's a ... threatening and ... (T: Yes.) overpowering ... (T: Yes.) and I want to keep it away from me. (T: Hm.) Like being scared of losing something, I don't know. (T: Mhm.) Plunging in too far and ...

T96: Hm. Yes. Losing your identity?

The therapist does an empathic guessing.

C97: Right. (T: Hm, yes.) Yeah, losing the 'me' in it.

T97: Yes. So, to protect yourself, you have to push away.

C98: That's what I want to do.

T98: Oh, that's what you want to do: Push away.

144

C99: Mm, but sometimes I feel . . . sucked in.

T99: Yes, yes . . . sometimes you felt: 'I didn't push away' (C: Right.), 'I let me suck in.' OK, yes, I see. And then, you have that awful feeling of losing your . . . 'you'. (C: Yes.) OK, yes, I . . . I know what you are feeling.

The therapist brings together different elements of the experience of the client. It's a moment of an experiential shift in the therapist, immediately followed by a deep shift in the client in C100.

C100: It's scary (starts crying).

T100: That's scary, losing 'yourself'.

C101: Yes. Hm, hm. (weeps)

T101: You're also sad about having lost yourself or . . . what's happening . . . now?

C102: It's hurting.

T102: It hurts, oh yeah.

C103: It's . . . painful. (T: Yeah.) Losing connection (T: Hmhm.), it's painful (sighs and weeps).

T103: Hm, you have had a lot of hurt and pain about this losing connection . . . Yeah, yeah.

During this fundamental breakthrough of the deeper meaning of the pain, the therapist restrains herself to empathic support and staying with the client in pain. Although the experience is painful, it brings a clear physical relief in the client. The meaning of the scary feeling is reconstituted and the client has regained the capacity to interact with experiences without being overwhelmed.

C104: Yes. (T: Mhm.) (weeps, sighs heavily)
(25 second silence)
And there is a lot of warmth I experience too.

After having received the felt meaning, the client feels ready for more. The self-motivated 'carrying forward' process takes the form of a continued self-exploration.

Up until here the session took 30 minutes. It continued for another 30 minutes, unfolding other important meanings.


## CODA

One year later, when the therapist asked the client for permission to use the recording for teaching purposes, the client wrote about this session: 'The work that was done together was very useful to me as it facilitated the process of getting in touch with painful feelings from the past which needed to be released. They were released one year ago, and since then I believe I have grown as a person. Therefore, I am happy and pleased that you should want to use the session. I think it would help to further the aims and understanding of person-centred psychotherapy.'

Therapy is a relational process of development, where focusing comes in when client and therapist pay attention inwardly to that unclear sense of something there. Many client-centred therapists don't have trouble with focusing as an inwardly arising process in the client, but they have trouble with the therapist 'teaching' that process. If the therapist rigidly follows the steps, there is a problem. However if the therapist gives precedence to the Rogerian attitudes and follows wherever the client takes her, bringing in the focusing attitude and integrating bits of the steps when the client gets stuck may make a wonderful difference.

REFERENCES

CORNELL, W. A. (1991), 'Too close/too distant: toward a typology of focusing process'. Paper presented at the Second International Conference on Client-Centred and Experiential Psychotherapy, University of Stirling, Scotland.

GENDLIN, E. T. (1981), *Focusing* (rev. ed.). New York: Bantam Books.

GREENBERG, L., RICE, L., and ELLIOTT, R. (in press). *Facilitating Emotional Change: a process-experiential approach.*

LEIJSSEN, M. (1990), 'On focusing and the necessary conditions of therapeutic personality change', in G. Lietaer, J. Rombauts and R. Van Balen (eds.), *Client-Centered and Experiential Psychotherapy in the Nineties.* Leuven: Leuven University Press.

PROUTY, G. F. (1990), 'Pre-therapy: theoretical evolution in the person-centered/experiential psychotherapy of schizophrenia and retardation', in G. Lietaer, J. Rombauts and R. Van Balen (eds.), op. cit.

## · 7 ·

# Looking In, Looking Out: Using Multi-Media Approaches in Person-Centred Therapy

### CAROLINE BEECH

## INTRODUCTION

As a person-centred therapist, I am increasingly using a variety of expressive media in my work. These include painting, visualization, body-focused work, movement, clay work and spatial work. My work is with individuals and with groups. Many of my clients are women who have difficulties around food, eating and body image.

In this chapter I will explore some of the learnings which have resulted from my work. In particular I will highlight the spatial aspects of the different modes of working, and their appropriateness to different therapeutic situations. This will be concentrated in a discussion of the possibilities for creating closeness or distance between the client and the material being described. I will list guidelines which I feel are appropriate to work of this type.

## BEGINNINGS

Several years ago when I was training as a therapist, I had a client whom I shall call Jane. On our second session Jane arrived with a book of guided fantasy exercises. She carried on bringing the book session after session. Initially the book caused me considerable dismay. I would explain that I was training in the person-centred approach, and so was not allowed to be directive. I would

148

empathize with her desire to work with fantasy and her horror at the silences which inevitably arose during our sessions. For weeks we battled on. Each session she would bring her book of fantasies, and each week I would make empathic reflections of her desire to be directed, discomfort at having to just talk, and frustration at my lack of co-operation.

Fortunately Jane was somewhat more persistent than I was. After some weeks it became obvious to me that we were not getting very far. Perhaps had my skills been better I would have found a way to put her at ease with my methods, but as it was she won me over to hers.

From that time things began to improve. I had run relaxation classes, so found no difficulty in helping her to relax while I read the fantasies from the book she had brought. Things might have stopped at that point, but I had a sense that more was possible. I also sensed that the fantasies which the book prescribed were not particularly relevant to Jane. So after a few weeks, I began to watch Jane's responses more closely. I began to notice that at times she seemed to be entering totally into the scene.

'It looks as if you have a sense of being somewhere,' I said. 'Can you say what's going on?' Jane's response was to describe a scene from her childhood. She was in a room in the house she had grown up in, her father standing in front of her. Her fear was evident as she faced him. With encouragement she spoke to him, raising unresolved issues which had stood between them since childhood.

We discussed the experience, and decided to continue working in a similar way. Over the year that we worked together, Jane and I learned many things about how it was possible to work. Often we would start with a fantasy from the book, but invariably we would end up in a new imagined world. Some of the scenes were recognizably regressive (Brazier, 1992), others were symbolic. Sometimes Jane would simply describe what she saw, but more often she would interact with the people she met. In those sessions she confronted people who had hurt her in the past, faced situations that she feared, and surrounded herself with images of how the future might be. Mostly the work was in her head, but sometimes we would play out scenes in the room, using whatever cushions or items of furniture there were to represent figures from her past.

My experience of working with Jane led me to question some of the assumptions I had made about my approach to therapy. Was it more empathic to follow Jane's need for structure or to insist on working in the style which I was learning? It also led me to consider ways of working which I had previously considered outside my field of work.

Since that time I have used a wide range of expressive and explorative techniques both with individuals and with groups. Sometimes the move into other media is initiated by a client. More often I now offer modes of working where they seem appropriate.

## IMAGES AND MEDIA

As I spend my time listening to others something which often strikes me is the clarity of images which both the client and myself can experience during therapy sessions. I am also struck by the power of these images to bring healing. Gendlin (1981) speaks of the shift which occurs when a person fully experiences their 'felt-sense' of a situation. My experience is that this felt-sense can generally be expressed in terms of an image.

The word 'image' used in this context may be interpreted in broad terms as something experienced by the client or therapist which has a representational quality. Images generally have a visual element to them, but may not be experienced primarily in that way. Images may be rooted in memory; scenes from the past. They may be real or imagined places. They may also be symbolic representations of the felt-sense. They may also be perceived as verbal, sometimes a single word, but if this is the case, they will have a meaning beyond the literal. An image is something that has the power to hold the attention beyond the immediate context of the therapy session. It may be a simple picture or may be a longer experiencing which alters over time, such as the reliving of a past event.

Images may occur spontaneously during the session. A client, whom I shall call John, in talking about a situation from the past, would suddenly begin to speak more quietly and seem to become smaller in the chair. My sense was that he was re-experiencing the feelings that he had as a child. If asked 'How old do you feel now?' he would often, sometimes with surprise, pinpoint an age without a second thought.

For the client in this situation, it would seem that two levels of operation are occurring. On one level the client is telling a story. On another level the image is beginning to form. The question asked by the therapist allows the client to respond spontaneously from the imaging part of himself. This serves to strengthen the image.

Thus, by responding to the imaging part of the client, the therapist helps the client to move from the interacting part of himself into the imaging one. This process might also be seen as hearing the client on a deeper level, or responding to the felt-sense behind the story.

So far I have described two scenarios in which image work may be introduced. The first, Jane's case, was a deliberate request to work in this way, the second, John's, an amplification of the client's spontaneous process. As I have become more aware of imagery in my work, I have offered clients ways of working which have further developed the imagery arising in the sessions. These methods have allowed us to work with images in new ways. They have also made the client's images more accessible, either by amplifying or by containing them. The possibility for amplification or containment of the client's experiencing of a felt-sense through the use of different media is central to this work.


AMPLIFICATION

Often clients speak of situations with detachment. It may be that their story is one that they have recounted many times. It may be that they have ceased to expect that anyone will really hear their distress. It may be that they have long since forgotten their own distress.

Some techniques which I use in my work seem particularly to help clients retrace the paths to these deeply buried parts of their experience, sometimes through regressive reliving of past events, often through more abstract images of half-acknowledged feelings. Such reconnection with the felt element in the story is an essential aspect of many therapeutic approaches (Rogers, Gendlin, Scheff etc.). In particular it is those techniques which help the client to focus within her own body which open up such pathways. This body awareness is very similar in function to the focusing techniques developed by Gendlin (1981). Indeed many of the suggestions which a therapist using focusing techniques might use in the sessions are similar to those which I might use.

In addition to body awareness, the client may also explore internal imagery. This image work can be similar to guided fantasy work of Jungian active imagination, and is directed by the client. In this work the therapist is outside the image, whilst the client holds it within herself.

Imagery of this kind may often provide a bridge to images which spill into the space of the therapy room. With these the client not only experiences the felt-sense within herself, but also surrounds herself with the image world. The therapist may then enter into the imaged world as companion. We may on occasion notice this externalization of imagery occurring spontaneously within the session. A client speaks angrily of his father, and glances towards the door as if expecting him to enter at any moment.

Such cues give the therapist a sense of the client's spatial construction of the image. For the therapist who is sensitive to such cues, a response may be to acknowledge the image, and the fact that it is being seen: 'You are looking over there, and I sense that you see your father.' Such a response is likely to have the effect of strengthening the client's image. As in the example given earlier, an image which was on the edge of perception becomes more focused. This process can be amplified further if the therapist asks the client to describe what he sees: his father's stance, his clothing, his surroundings; a process reminiscent of scene setting in psycho-drama (Moreno, 1987). From such a beginning, therapist and client may move into an imagined world, represented in the space of the room.

The externalization of the image world offers new fields of exploration to the client. Anchored in the space of the therapy room, aspects of the image can be safely put aside whilst others are explored to the full. The client may leave his own place in the image and experience the world and himself through his father's eyes, sure in the knowledge that he may return to his own perspective when he wishes. The possibilities for dialogue, exploration, expression of feelings, and sharing of experience are limited only by the imagination of client and therapist.

## CONTAINMENT

Whilst the activities described so far will generally help clients to gain more contact with their felt-sense of an issue, there are times when the client feels overwhelmed by the experience (Cornell, 1991). He or she may feel unable to look at the material at all, but also feel blocked from exploring other areas of life.

Where this is the case, some media offer ways of working which place the image outside the client. This enables the person to face the experience or feeling which was so terrifying, seeing it, but keeping a safe distance from it. It also enables an image to be viewed in its entirety. Interrelationships can be seen, and connections made.

This externalization of the client's image world can be achieved through fantasy work in which the client places herself outside the image, as observer of a scene, a process akin to watching a film. More frequently it is achieved through the use of arts media.

The sense of containment which is achieved through painting can allow powerful expression of feelings which might otherwise be overwhelming to the client. Pictures may take on a quality which incorporates this power. Joy Schaverien (Schaverien, 1992) perceives this quality as a form of transference. She also describes the transformation of a picture into a scapegoat, having the power to rid the client of the bad feelings which it represents.

Certainly it is noticeable that some clients will deliberately destroy their painting at the end of a session, whilst others will be keen to preserve it in some way, either keeping it themselves or entrusting it to the therapist. This concern highlights the symbolic nature of paintings as artefacts and containers, which is additional to their symbolism as images.

## SPACE AND MULTI-MEDIA WORK

In considering an integrative approach to multi-media work, space provides a useful focus. When we consider the spatial aspect of this work, it becomes clear that there are three elements within the therapeutic relationship: the therapist, the client and the material, which can stand in different spatial relationships to each other. Different modes of working allow different interrelationships.

Three basic spatial combinations occur. The first basic position in which the client experiences the working material within herself is typical of focusing and body oriented therapies. In this case the therapist is outside the material and the client inside, or at least contains it within a part of her body space.

Such material frequently originates from a bodily feeling. An image develops which may seem to the client contained within her body, or surrounding her. Its focus remains with the client, and does not become externally fixed in the fabric of the therapy room. Such an experiencing of the material can be extremely powerful both in giving insight, and in bringing about catharsis. It may also feel overwhelming. It is experienced by the client as being with her alone. The therapist is merely observer and commentator.

The second positioning is that in which the client externalizes the material, giving it a location within the therapy room which has a spatial fixity. This is likely to happen in sculpting, gestalt, or psychodramatically based work. In this instance therapist and client may both be located inside the material, but, because the material has been given a spatial existence separate from the client, it is possible for both therapist and client to move about within it, and even move outside it. Such movement permits material to be viewed from many angles. It permits one area to be explored in depth, without the client feeling the need to retain a hold on other areas.

One example of this may occur when a client is aware of contradictory feelings towards another person. This client may choose to use two chairs to represent these contradictory facets which she perceives in the other – 'This is the mother who I feel loved by, and this is the one who I felt neglected by as a child.' By giving the two aspects separate locations, the client is able to then move on and explore feelings related to each separately, knowing that the other feelings have not been lost, and that they may be returned to at any time. The client may also choose to view each facet from a number of directions: in confrontation, from alongside or within, from the distant position of an outsider, from the position of another family member, or even the position of the other facet of the person – 'How does the loving mother feel about the neglectful one?'

The third instance, found in painting and other arts based work, places the material outside the client, on paper, or some other object. Here both therapist and client may observe, hold, or enter into dialogue with the material, but may not enter into it. The material is contained. This quality of containment can offer important therapeutic advantages. Material which has been internal, part of self, becomes external, an object. In this new location it can be seen in new ways.

In recent work one client described a weight inside his chest. He was unable to get any sense of what the weight might be, and felt overwhelmed by it whenever he tried to get more in touch with it. When I suggested he use paints to explore the feeling, he painted a large black object floating in a green sea. This painting became the focus for the remainder of the session. Being able to look at the object he had painted and see its extent and its surroundings took away some of the fear that had overwhelmed him when we

155

had tried to explore it earlier. It was possible to identify the grief which it contained, and the isolation which surrounded it.

This third spatial relationship may also be important in offering an overview. Another client who had spent several sessions talking about different incidents from her life used drawing to produce a map from her birth to the present. By marking the incidents across the page, new connections emerged. She began to become more aware of not only the repeating patterns of losses which had occurred in her life, but also of the important relationships which had emerged time and again and brought her out of the pain which she was enduring.

So, different spatial combinations allow very different experiencing of the material which is explored in therapy. In multi-media work, the therapist and client may use different media at different times in order to explore different facets of the same material. We may think of the use of different media as something akin to the use of a zoom lens on a camera, which has a range from wide-angle to telephoto. At some times the client may need to take in a wide field of vision, whilst at others the client needs to be able to look at some area in minute close-up. Different media provide this possibility for the client.

To go beyond this analogy, however, different media offer other possibilities, as the client may not only choose to view, but also to enter into material, and move around within it, thus gaining many different perspectives. We may stand in our familiar position, or we may move and see the world from our partner's or mother's or child's position.

A further important spatial aspect which is often evident in the work is that the externalizing of the material creates a new way of relating for therapist and client. As the material being explored in the sessions becomes more tangibly represented, therapist and client may find themselves joining together in a journey of exploration. They may jointly view material from a distance, or enter into the different elements of it. Their relationship becomes a partnership. Conventionally therapists and clients sit opposite one another. In multi-media work it is common for therapist and client to be side by side. This 'alongside' experience is also felt at a deeper level. Sessions more literally become a shared exploration of the client's experiencing.

## COMBINING DIFFERENT MODES OF WORKING

So far this has discussed different modes of working separately. However perhaps the most important aspect of multi-media work is the opportunity which it provides to combine and juxtapose different modes of working. Exploration in one mode leads naturally into another and another. Each gives a different view, a new perspective. Visualization can move into art, which in turn can move into a playing-out in the therapy room. Once the scene is mapped, the client may use focusing technique to explore each part of the image in turn.

One client spent the first part of her session painting what appeared to be a rainbow with concentric coloured arches. Having done this she surveyed her work, and described it articulately as the map of her life to date. She saw it as a tunnel stretching back towards her birth.

At this point I suggested that we should map out the tunnel in the room, so together we designated a line from one end of the room to the other with zones of colour as they had been on the rainbow, but this time set out as stripes of imagined colour. The immediate shift which occurred for the client was one of awe at the prospect of being within the rainbow, rather than regarding it from a distance. Having achieved a sense of the whole, we were then able to explore individual parts of the tunnel by physically visiting them. In each there was the opportunity to re-experience the inner sense of that period of the client's life through body-focused regression. Some scenes became extremely vivid, and the woman became intensely emotional, but my sense was that she always retained a sense of the whole, and of the possibility of moving into another area.

One purple zone, however, remained untouched. Although the

woman expressed feelings of wanting to visit it, she also had a fear of being overwhelmed by it. We tried using painting to explore what might be within that area, but she had the sense of needing to actually stand in it in order to exorcize its power over her. To do so, the reminder of the whole span of the rainbow needed to be more tangible. She needed to be able, literally, to hold on to another part of her past in order to reassure herself that this purple area was not all-consuming; that life had existed beyond it. We achieved entry into this fearful area by creating a lifeline; a strand of thread of another colour that she could take with her into the darkness. It ceased to be overwhelming for her. Though the area still held fears and pain, she now recognized that it had limits. It became possible for her to hold on to a sense of other times while she re-experienced the terror of that time.

It has been my experience that it is often the shift between media which provides new insight. Speaking gives an insight into the client's process through one window; other media provide different windows. Thus, by shifting our perspective, we may gain new insights. But the effects of changing medium seem to go beyond a simple change of perspective. It often seems as if the shift itself provokes change or insight. In the example which I have just given, we can recognize a number of phases. An initial cognitive mapping out of the whole, containing within it the seeds of a number of emotive memories, represented by the different colours, whose choice may have depended upon a mix of conscious and unconscious factors. A shift into the spatial dimension brought an immediate sense of scale that had not been present in the painting. This is a lifetime. It fills the therapy room. It is greater than can be captured in a few brush strokes. Later, shifts into the body brought an intensification of experience. The almost magical effect of the coloured thread in the final part illustrates the magical talisman qualities with which objects within the scene are often invested.

Shifts of insight may also occur within a particular medium through a shift in position. This can be seen very clearly in psychodrama where the technique of role reversal can allow the protagonist to gain insight instantaneously into another's perspective, by taking their spatial position. Such a technique need not be confined to groups. It can also be achieved through spatial allocation within the therapy room, for example using chairs, but can also be used in guided fantasy work.

We can also see from this example that the progression from one medium to another can provide a means of control for the client who is overwhelmed by feelings arising from the issues which he is discussing. If a containing medium, such as painting, is used first, the client may then feel more confident to explore the feelings in other ways, having some sense of their extent. Similarly if the client feels chaotic and confused, to produce a visible image can focus thoughts and feelings, and provide a map or sense of direction.

Multi-media work provides not one, but several media. The combining of different ways of working produces a style of therapy which offers more than its individual components. The process whereby combining different media appears to offer something which is more productive than any of the media used singly is one that is also observed by Natalie Rogers, who comments on the importance of the actual act of integration, as being separate from and additional to the separate therapeutic effects of different expressive techniques used individually: '. . . The excitement in me is about integrating all of the above [modes of working] and finding that it is something more than any one of those modes' (N. Rogers, 1990). Central to this is the release of creativity which arises when a series of media are used. Such creativity seems to be associated with new insights. It also goes beyond insight, becoming the spark which may enable growth of new potential.

## MULTI-MEDIA WORK AND THE THERAPEUTIC RELATIONSHIP

The extent to which the use of different media within the therapeutic setting affects the relationship between therapist and client must be an important consideration, given the centrality of that relationship to the whole therapy process.

One factor in this work which makes it distinctive is the externalization of the client's material so that it may become an object within the therapy room. Whilst this material element, the 'content' of the session, is present in conventional 'talking' therapy, in multi-media work it is often tangibly in the room. This strong presence of the therapeutic material as separate from the client allows therapist and client to enter into an exploration which can have an enhanced feeling of partnership. As has already been pointed out, the physical positioning of the therapist alongside the client may also lend symbolic support to this shift in the relationship towards equality.

Conversely there are a number of changes in the style of response of the therapist which may lend a more directive style to the therapist's relationship with the client. As such, the relevance of equality may be more questionable.

The therapist in multi-media work may use a large number of questions. The use of questions in person-centred therapy is contentious. Rogers used very few direct questions. The general effect of a question is to encourage the client to think. Often questions have the effect of extending the field of information gathered, but decreasing the depth of the interaction. In multi-media work there are times when this effect is desirable, as with psychodrama, where setting the scene before the action, deepens the protagonist's experience (Brazier, 1991). Psychodrama uses questions to extend the protagonist's visual sense of the environment being created, and develop the identities of characters being played by auxiliaries. In multi-media work they may fulfil a similar function.

Questions in multi-media work are a response to empathic understanding, and may be invitations to extend the felt sense of the situation. This may be done by asking the client to develop the visual image, as in the example just quoted, or to get a deeper sense of what it signifies. Elfie Hinterkopf writes of the value of questions to the focuser (Hinterkopf, 1992). 'Asking' is the fifth step in the process developed by Gendlin for teaching focusing (Gendlin, 1981). Hinterkopf states that besides speeding up the process, 'The asking step keeps me from "spacing out" or wandering . . . I have found when I use only the Being With instructions and omit the

Asking step, I often feel confused and lost as though I am swimming in a fog. When the questions are asked in a friendly, gentle, patient way, they invite me to stay with my felt sense and to see what comes.'

My sense is that both these points apply to multi-media work in which participants are deeply involved in their own imagery. It seems that empathic reflection can leave the person in the fog, whilst a tentative question can sometimes help that fog to clear.

Some questions may have an interrupting quality. At times this may also be important if the therapist is to keep close contact with the client. For the client who is experiencing a regressed state, for instance, the therapist may need to ask directly 'How old do you feel?' in order for the client to gain awareness of her regression. Such a question can often prompt a spontaneous shift into a scene from childhood.

At times the therapist may take on a teaching or guiding role. The client may need direction to gain sufficient relaxation in order to enter into an image. He may need prompting to explore body-based feelings. He may need alternative ways of working suggested, or the explanation of techniques such as role reversal or sculpting.

Where these different functions are performed by the therapist, some prefer a separation from the main therapeutic session. Focusers working as therapists frequently prefer to send clients to learn focusing skills from others in workshops. I have myself suggested psychodrama or bodywork groups to clients on occasion. Such separation of the teaching of techniques from the actual therapy session can be useful and appropriate, not least in offering the client new experience of working with others in a group context. In my experience, however, it is not always necessary.

For me congruence is an important element in sharing a different skill or technique: 'I don't know if this will work for you, but I have often found drawing a map of different events in my life a useful way of getting an overview of things – it feels as if you're trying to do something similar, and I'm wondering if putting it on paper might help.'

It feels important to me that the therapist is aware of the

limitations and arbitrary element in the choices of techniques offered. Whatever theoretical construct she uses, the final choice can only ever be an estimation of what may be appropriate. Practicalities such as availability of materials, the therapist's own interests, creativity and experience, time factors and other non-therapeutic elements may all play a part in influencing the choice of medium offered. The therapist needs to be willing to offer possibilities with openness, and be ready to respond empathically to the client's reaction.

A third major shift in the therapist/client relationship may involve an increase in the level of dependency felt by the client for the therapist, either in short or long term. This may result from the increased directiveness shown by the therapist, but may also be a function of the regressive nature of some multi-media work. It may also be that as the client enters more experientially into the frightening areas of his life, he feels a need for the therapist's presence, providing a link with the day-to-day world that he has temporarily left.

The issue of dependency is a complex one. Some therapeutic models regard it as a normal part of therapy to be encouraged as a stage in the process. In the person-centred world such a deliberate courting of the client's dependent or childlike parts is generally avoided. It is not my intention to do more than raise this debate here, but it does seem important that any therapist using different media be aware that certain styles of interaction, such as more directive or overtly supportive, regressive or cathartic work may be more likely to encourage dependency.

## CREATING GUIDELINES FOR MULTI-MEDIA WORK

In the previous section of this chapter, a number of qualities have been identified which may be present in the therapeutic relationship which uses multi-media approaches. A multi-media approach is not necessarily intrinsically different from other person-centred work in these respects, but does require a particular sensitivity to issues of power and boundaries.

The use of the wider space of the therapy room opens many possibilities. The therapist may move into the client's world more literally than is possible in verbal therapeutic encounters. The potential for intrusion is therefore greater. In view of this potential for intrusion there do seem to be certain boundaries that the therapist needs to maintain.

This section attempts to clarify some guidelines which a person-centred therapist using different media may wish to adhere to.

1. *Empathic connection*: The first essential for any therapist venturing into new media is the maintenance of the empathic connection. A prerequisite of this is that, even when suggesting a new mode of expression, the therapist maintains a following position. The suggestion should be a response to the client's process, and should be offered with the same willingness for rejection as any other empathic response.

2. *Explicit congruence with regard to the process*: Wherever possible therapists should share their own thoughts about the process of the therapy, and choices of working mode. Multi-media approaches work best where therapist and client maintain a relationship as companions on the therapeutic journey.

3. *Respect for spatial fixities*: As the client allocates image identities to locations or objects within the room, care needs to be taken that these identities are respected. Such objects will retain an element of identity even after the image world has apparently been dismantled. In general the client may wish to perform any physical dismantling herself.

4. *Maintaining a neutral position*: In my experience in individual therapy it is generally inappropriate for the therapist to deliberately take on a role other than her own. To do so would risk leaving the client alone in an imagined world. This is not to say that transfer-

ence does not on occasions occur spontaneously, but when this happens the therapist's primary role is 'to understand and accept' (Rogers, 1951, p. 203).

5. *Recognizing the multi-layered quality of images*: Images are representations of the felt sense. As such they are both themselves, memories or pictures, and metaphoric resonances of present thoughts and feelings. For an image to occur, there will be a live element in the client's life which is symbolically represented by the image. In working with images, the therapist must be willing to move with fluidity between different representations. The therapist must also be able to recognize the symbolic quality of the work, and must be at ease working with material that is not necessarily immediately comprehensible in a rational way. The image has a logic of its own.

6. *Reaching closure*: The ending of any image-based work is important. Sometimes, if the journey has had a number of steps, the path may need to be retraced. There may be things that need to be said or done at some stages. There may need to be time for silent contemplation and reorientation, or discussion of the experience. It may be risky for a client who has been re-experiencing himself as a five-year-old to go straight out to his car and drive home! In general the client will have a sense of what stages of closure he needs. It is the therapist's task to be sure that time is allowed and an invitation to finish appropriately is given.

## SUMMARY

I have outlined some aspects of the work which I am doing as a therapist using different arts media. Multi-media work has much in common with expressive and experiential therapies. It is not something radically different or new. On the other hand, it does offer some new perspectives for integrating different modes of working into the person-centred approach.

In particular this chapter has offered a theoretical framework which explores the spatial relationship between therapist, client, and the subject matter of therapy. It offers insight into the different interrelationships of these three elements which can be achieved through different modes of working. Finally, it explores the effects of these different styles of working upon the therapeutic relationship itself. The work is in a state of constant review and discovery. Its process of evolution is in itself a creative journey.

REFERENCES

BRAZIER, D. (1991), *A Guide to Psychodrama*. London: Association for Humanistic Psychology.

BRAZIER, D. (1992), *Our Many Lives*. Newcastle: Eigenwelt Interskill.

CORNELL, A. W. (1991), *Too close/too distant*. Paper presented at the Second International Conference on Client-Centred and Experiential Psychotherapy, University of Stirling, Scotland.

GENDLIN, E. (1981), *Focusing*. New York: Bantam.

GENDLIN, E. (1990), 'The small steps of the therapy process: how they come and how to help them come', in G. Lietaer, J. Rombauts and R. Van Balen (eds.), *Client-Centred and Experiential Psychotherapy in the Nineties*, pp. 205–24. Leuven, Belgium: Leuven University Press.

HINTERKOPF, E. (1992), 'In favour of the asking step', *The Focusing Connection*, 9, 3, p. 5.

MORENO, J. (1987), in J. Fox (ed.), *The Essential Moreno*. New York: Springer.

ROGERS, C. (1951), *Client-Centred Therapy*. London: Constable.

ROGERS, C. (1961), *On Becoming a Person*. London: Constable.

ROGERS, C. (1978), *On Personal Power*. London: Constable.

ROGERS, C. (1980), *A Way of Being*. Boston: Houghton Mifflin.

ROGERS, C. (1983), *Freedom to Learn for the 80s*. Columbus, Ohio: Merrill.

ROGERS, C. (1986), 'A client-centred/person-centred approach to therapy', in H. Kirschenbaum and V. Henderson (eds.), *The Carl Rogers Reader*, pp. 135–57). London: Constable.

ROGERS, N. (1985), *The Creative Connection: a person-centred approach to expressive therapy*. Santa Rosa, California: The Person-Centered Expressive Therapy Institute.

SCHAVERIEN, J. (1992), *The Revealing Image*. London: Routledge.

# · 8 ·

# Teaching Focusing with Five Steps and Four Skills

## ANN WEISER CORNELL

### BACKGROUND

Focusing was first described in 1964 (by Gendlin) as a process of attending to and carrying forward something directly felt but not yet clear. It was a description of a naturally occurring, unprompted client process associated with successful outcomes in psychotherapy.

Soon researchers moved beyond observation of the process to teaching the process. 'Now that we can define the sort of interview behavior which eventuates in success, it no longer seems right to let failure-predicted modes of behavior simply continue ... We have embarked on a new avenue of research, in which we will attempt to "teach" this "focusing" manner of process to clients' (Gendlin, Beebe, Cassens, Klein, and Oberlander, 1968).

Published with this 1968 paper was a 'Focusing Manual', that is, a set of instructions to be read to a client who silently followed the instructions. Client reports afterward helped the researchers determine whether focusing occurred.

The following excerpt is from this 1968 Focusing Manual:

Just to yourself, inside you, I would like you to pay attention to a very special part of you. Pay attention to that part where you usually feel sad, glad, or scared ...

See what comes to you when you ask yourself, 'How am I now?' 'How do I feel?' 'What is the main thing for me right

167

now?' Let it come, in whatever way it comes to you, and see how it is.

If among the things that you have just thought about, there was a major personal problem which felt important, continue with it. Otherwise, select a meaningful personal problem to think about . . .

Pay attention there where you usually feel things, and in there you can get a sense of what all the problem feels like. Let yourself feel all of that . . .

Now take what is fresh, or new, in the feel of it now . . . Just as you feel it, try to find some new words or pictures to capture what your present feeling is all about . . .

If the words or pictures that you now have make some fresh difference, see what that is. Let the words or pictures change until they feel just right in capturing your feeling. (p. 239.)

It is noteworthy that in this first procedure for teaching focusing, the six steps familiar from Eugene Gendlin's popular book *Focusing* (1981) are not found. There is no Clearing a space, no Asking, no Receiving. The instructions can be related to the steps of Getting a felt sense, Getting a handle, and Resonating the handle, but barely resemble them as they are now taught. Elsewhere in the same paper, focusing is described as having four 'phases': 1. Direct reference, 2. Referent movement, 3. Wide application, and 4. Content mutation. These are nothing like the six steps developed later.

When I encountered Gendlin's teaching in 1972–4, he was using focusing instructions quite like the 1968 version, but with some new aspects. One evening he led us in an exercise that, in retrospect, I recognize as Clearing a space. (It used the metaphor of peeking into bundles and setting them down.) Steps were not mentioned as such.

Sometime between 1974 and 1978 when the first edition of *Focusing* was published, the six steps were specified. Linda Prier recalls (personal communication) attending focusing training groups with Eugene Gendlin in New York in 1976–77. She describes a teaching process that was in formation. 'We did setting out, finding a felt sense, getting a handle, and asking. Gene said that all the steps really applied all the time. He also said they could apply in any order.' Roger Levin recalls (personal communication) that, at that same time, around 1976, 'The steps process was developing. There was some confusion about whether there were five or six steps. Rechecking the handle [later called Resonating the handle] was the one that sometimes was included and sometimes wasn't.' Gene Gendlin remembers (personal communication) that Receiving was the step that was added last.

Clearly there was a continual evolution of focusing teaching, up until the publication of *Focusing* in 1978. After 1978 the picture is markedly different. Nearly every author describing focusing has used six steps, usually exactly the same six steps. (They are: Clearing a space, Getting a felt sense, Getting a handle, Resonating the handle, Asking and Receiving.) A German book about focusing, *Dein Körper weiss die Antwort* (Siems, 1986) uses the same six steps. Mia Leijssen (1990), in her insightful paper in the Belgium conference volume, lists the six steps, with slight differences, even though in many other ways her paper challenges those who have a static view of focusing. The exception to this is Edwin McMahon and Peter Campbell, currently the most influential teachers of focusing in the United States other than Gene Gendlin, who teach different steps. Their book (1985) lists five: 1. Finding a space by taking an inventory, 2. Feeling which one is number one, 3. Is it OK to be with this?, 4. Letting go into it, 5. Allowing it to express itself. Interestingly, they have since added an ending step, so they are now also teaching six steps (personal communication).

Led perhaps by this near universal acceptance of the six steps, many authors fall into what I consider an error, and say 'focusing has six steps' rather than 'in teaching focusing it is helpful to use six steps'. Gendlin himself may have added to this confusion, for despite declarations in workshops that the steps were to be used only for teaching the process, not as a description of the process itself, he wrote in *Focusing*, 'The inner act of focusing can be broken down into six main subacts or movements' (p. 43).

169

To me it makes sense that, in developing our teaching of a complex person-centred process like focusing, there would continue to be an evolution in our understanding of which formulation of steps is the clearest and most easily taught description of the process. I believe it would even be helpful for there to be different sets of teaching steps in use by different teachers, because when students are encouraged to work with different teachers, they then see clearly that the process is more than the steps. There might even be a way of teaching that goes beyond steps.

For the last few years I have been experimenting with a method of teaching focusing with five steps and four skills, with notable success. Students of focusing, students of focusing teaching, and other focusing teachers have all told me that this method is easy to understand and to do. A high percentage of focusing students report that focusing continues to be a part of their lives after the class, which I consider to be the most desirable outcome.

The division into 'steps' and 'skills' is based on a realization that some aspects of focusing need to come in a particular order ('steps'), while other aspects are brought in either globally or as needed throughout the session ('skills'). Previously, in working with steps alone, I kept finding myself explaining that, for example, although Resonating was the fourth step, it actually came at any part of the session where it was needed. Since I have been teaching in terms of steps and skills, the amount of 'yes-but-not-really' type of explaining has decreased considerably.

## THE FIVE STEPS

In my model of the focusing process, I use five teaching steps that describe the parts of the focusing process that are always there, that come one after the other, in order. Currently, they are:

1. Bringing awareness into the body
2. Finding or inviting a felt sense

3. Getting a handle
4. Being with
5. Ending

## BRINGING AWARENESS INTO THE BODY

Bringing awareness into the body is implied in Gendlin's steps, but seems to 'go without saying'. I prefer to say it, because I have seen beginning focusing students get in their own way by forgetting to bring awareness into the body as the very first step of focusing. This step serves as a reminder to bring awareness especially into the middle area of the body: throat, chest, stomach, abdomen – because felt senses typically (though not always) come there. For Too Distant people (Cornell, 1991) especially, this step is worth taking time with, as well as for people who meditate and need grounding in the body for focusing to be successful. But all focusers start this way, even if they don't need to take much time with it. Contrast this first step with the commonly taught first step of Clearing a space, which most experienced focusers treat as optional.

## FINDING OR INVITING A FELT SENSE

Once awareness is in the body, people typically have one or two types of experience. One is to discover that there is a felt sense already there, perhaps something that has been calling for attention already. ('Yes, there's a tightness in my stomach; I've been feeling it all day.') The other is that the middle of the body may be feeling fairly clear and open when awareness is first brought there, but that a felt sense can come there if invited. This invitation may involve saying something like, 'How am I now?' or 'What in my life feels like it needs attention?' To reflect these two types of process, I have changed the name of this step from Getting a felt sense to Finding or inviting a felt sense.

GETTING A HANDLE

In name and procedure this step is like Gendlin's. It involves finding a word, or words, or an image, or a sound or a gesture, to describe, fit, or match the feel of the felt sense. Notice how appropriate the order is here. A felt sense is found or invited, then a description is found for how it feels. It couldn't be the other way around!

BEING WITH

This is a renaming of Gendlin's step five, called Asking. After getting the handle, the person spends time with the felt sense with an attitude of friendly, respectful curiosity. If necessary, an open-ended question is asked inwardly as a way of holding awareness there with interested curiosity. But the condition of inwardly spending time with the felt sense is more central to this step than the activity of asking questions, which is not needed in every process. In fact, calling this step Asking can mislead beginning focusers, because they may imagine that the felt sense must 'speak' in reply.

In observing the focusing process in experienced focusers, where little or no guiding is needed, I have noticed that quite often there are no questions involved in this phase of the process. Instead, meaning associated with the felt sense seems to simply flow forward. The asking of questions is an attempt to stimulate for the new focuser this flowing forth of 'more' that is found in the unprompted process. So the step is renamed Being with, with the understanding that asking questions may be part of it.

ENDING

Gendlin's steps don't mention the process of ending the session. His sixth step, Receiving, was not intended as an ending step, but is often understood that way by students because of its position as the sixth step. What seems to be helpful to people learning focusing is the inclusion of a special Ending step. In this step, the focuser marks the place as something that can be returned to at another time, and takes time to thank and appreciate what has come.

## THE FOUR SKILLS

I use the term 'the four skills' to describe the other key parts of the focusing process, which are used as needed throughout the process. At this time, they are:

Finding the right distance
Being friendly with what's there
Resonating
Receiving

### FINDING THE RIGHT DISTANCE

The skill of finding the right distance reflects the insight that people in Too Close process need the felt experience to be a little farther away, and people in Too Distant process need it to come a little closer. Once focusing students understand the concept of finding the right distance, they have a skill that is helpful whether they are in Too Close or Too Distant process. If focusing feels blocked, they can ask, 'Am I at the right distance from this?' If the answer is 'No,' they can call on techniques for setting something out, or for bringing it closer.

### BEING FRIENDLY WITH WHAT'S THERE

This skill captures the importance of the focuser's attitude toward his or her own felt experience. Focusing works best when the focuser's attitude toward what comes is accepting, open, respectful, like an understanding friend. The emphasis on this is evident in

Gendlin's work, but he did not make it a step. McMahon and Campbell did make it a step, called Is it OK to be with this? For me, it is a skill, because it is relevant at every point in the session.

## RESONATING

Resonating is the skill of checking back with the sense and getting the sense of rightness about what has come. Gendlin's step Resonating the handle comes directly after Getting a handle and before Asking. When teaching Resonating the handle, I kept having to explain that actually, resonating occurs all the way through, and many things other than the handle are resonated. Anything emerging in the process is checked back with the sense to see if it feels right. This helps impel the forward movement of the process, and helps the focuser stay grounded in the body.

## RECEIVING

Receiving is pausing to welcome and protect the new, fresh sense that comes with any felt shift, however large or small. This may occur at any point in the session. Even when first bringing awareness into the body, the focuser may become aware of something new and surprising, and even at that point it is important to do Receiving. Receiving is helpful as a way to gently encourage faint, delicate felt senses, and also to feel the many sides of a large, complex felt sense. It can serve as a 'pause' for focusers startled or overwhelmed by a felt shift. It is also a means of protecting the new sense from critics, analysers, go-getters, and other interfering inner characters.

## FOCUSING COURSE FORMAT

I'd like to offer a brief description of my focusing course format, because it has evolved along with the method of teaching steps and skills. (For more details, see Cornell, 1990b.)

The course format has three interrelated aspects:

1. Teaching focusing so that people are enabled to continue in focusing partnerships.
2. Introducing active listening at an early stage with an emphasis on helping the focuser 'resonate' his or her own words.
3. Teaching focusing as a process of 'self-guiding' so that learning focusing is equivalent to internalizing the guide.

### THE INDIVIDUAL SESSION

Students are strongly encouraged to start with a one-hour individual session. In this session, the teacher guides the student through the focusing process. (For more on the evolution of guiding see Cornell, 1991. For more on the specifics of guiding itself, see Cornell, 1990a.)

Starting with an individual session follows from the principle that each person has a uniquely right focusing process, and that it is important for each person to experience his or her own process before hearing generalizations which might be heard as prescriptions.

### THE FIRST CLASS MEETING

Classes are small, with no more than five students. At the first class meeting the teacher describes the history of focusing and the special concept of the felt sense. The group is guided together through an exercise in experiencing different felt senses. This is the only time that group guiding is done, and it is done only because in the first class people may be reluctant to focus individually.

After the students have reported what they want to report about their experiences in the exercise, the teacher describes the four skills. Students are asked to spend time at various times during the week sensing in their body, and no more.

## THE SECOND CLASS MEETING

The second class begins with an invitation to the students to report on their experiences during the week. Then the teacher describes the five steps. In the remaining time, each student is guided in focusing, for about twenty minutes each. We have found that twenty minutes is enough time to have a distinct focusing experience if Clearing a space is offered only as needed. Having had an individual session previously also seems to help students 'get something' in this class meeting in twenty minutes.

The other students are asked to watch the session for the steps and skills. They are also told that their respectful attention will help the session go well for the focuser.

Students are asked to set aside a time in the week between the classes and try focusing alone. They are also given a reading assignment for the next class, on focusing with a listener and listening to a focuser.

## THE THIRD CLASS MEETING

Students are first invited to share reports of their focusing experiences during the week. The teacher especially asks to hear trouble or blocks.

Next the teacher gives a short talk on the complementary roles of focusing and active listening. The emphasis is on teaching both sides of the interaction as skills: listening to a focuser and focusing with a listener. The listener is asked to respond with a reflection of some kind in every pause by the focuser. The focuser is asked to use the listener's reflection to resonate with his/her felt sense.

The teacher is the first focuser, and a student is the first listener. The listener is instructed to reflect only, and give no questions or suggestions. The teacher focuses, modelling self-guiding (see below) using the help of a listener. Ten minutes is taken, using a volunteer to keep time. After the interaction, each person says how it felt, starting with the listener. The observers are then invited to comment on the process, but no comments on the content are allowed.

The listener is invited to be the next focuser, and someone volunteers to be the next listener. The teacher is the last listener.

New listeners typically are amazed at the pleasure they felt at being able to concentrate on the focuser without feeling responsible for the process, yet they also comment that they felt as if they were not needed, or not helping. The focusers then typically respond that hearing the listening response was quite helpful, enabling them to stay on track, stay grounded, etc.


## THE FOURTH CLASS MEETING

The teacher begins with a presentation on blocks to focusing, describing typical blocks such as the internal critic, the need to find a solution, etc. Students then have another listening-focusing round robin, this time without the teacher taking a turn. Turns are longer, around fifteen minutes, and the focuser is urged to ask for help if she or he comes up against a block. The teacher steps in to help with guiding if asked, but otherwise the listener continues to do active listening as the process unfolds.

After each session, focusers discuss what they have learned about their own blocks that day and how they can respond when experiencing them.

## THE FIFTH CLASS MEETING

The teacher presents the concept of self-guiding, and explains that for the last two classes the students have been doing self-guiding; that is, they have been learning to guide themselves through focusing with the support of a listener who does not guide. The teacher goes over a list of the skills of self-guiding (e.g. 'Being able to bring awareness into the body'), and clears up remaining questions.

The teacher then goes over a list of guidelines for practice sessions, which give a simple structure that can be followed when there is no teacher. This is a distillation of the guidelines that the class has already been following for the last two class sessions. Special emphasis is placed on the guideline that says, 'The focuser can say how she or he wants to be listened to, both before and during the session.'

The students then have another listening-focusing round robin, with emphasis on this guideline. The listener is freed to respond less strictly, no longer having to reflect in every pause. The focuser is given the responsibility to say if she or he wants more or less reflection, or reflection of a different type. The teacher stays out of the interactions as much as possible, and lets the students give each other feedback.

At the very end of the class, the students are given lists with each other's names and addresses, and are encouraged to discuss meeting with each other, in pairs or larger groups, for further practice. They are also told how to contact the free practice groups ('Changes groups') that meet in the area.

## KEY ASPECTS OF THE CLASS FORMAT

The class design is based on observation of experienced focusers, who typically do not need guiding but are helped by reflection from a listener. Therefore, students are introduced as early as possible to the format of focusing with a listener. Experienced focusers also do not pay conscious attention to steps and skills as such; rather, focusing is experienced as a flow along an inner track. Students are encouraged to focus in this way as early as possible, with support offered to help with any blocks.

A primary goal is to teach focusing so that students are able to continue with it beyond the class. Since our experience has taught us that the vast majority of people who continue with focusing do so with the support of a focusing partnership or a focusing practice group, the teaching is aimed at readying the students for partnership and group practice. The last three class sessions are models of group practice, involving the teacher less and less. People whose aim it is to focus alone after the class are also helped by this format, because focusing alone requires internalizing an empathic non-judgemental listener, and the class practice facilitates this.

In all cases, the teaching is based on giving the focusers responsibility for their own process, including the power to request from the listener whatever help the focuser feels would be most facilitative.

## SUMMARY

Focusing is a naturally occurring, inwardly arising process associated with forward life movement. The description of this process for teaching is necessarily always an approximation. The steps and skills offered in this chapter are the best found by the author so far for communicating focusing to new learners. The phenomenon of focusing is there to be observed by every therapist and every focusing teacher. It is proposed that all focusing teaching be aimed at enabling the student or client to have access to this process easily, with minimal outside help, and each in his or her own way.

REFERENCES

CAMPBELL, PETER A., and MCMAHON, EDWIN M. (1985), *Biospirituality: focusing as a way to grow.* Chicago: Loyola University Press.

CORNELL, ANN WEISER (1990a), *A Guiding Manual*. Focusing Resources, 2625 Alcatraz Ave., 202, Berkeley, Ca 94705. Revised 1991.

CORNELL, ANN WEISER (1990b), 'How I teach people to focus with each other', *The Focusing Folio*, Vol. 9, 4. The Focusing Institute, 731 S. Plymouth Court, Suite 801, Chicago, Il 60605.

CORNELL, ANN WEISER (1991), 'Too close/too distant: toward a typology of focusing process.' Presented at the Second International Conference on Client-Centred and Experiential Psychotherapy, University of Stirling, Scotland.

GENDLIN, EUGENE (1964), 'A theory of personality change', in P. Worchel and D. Byrne (eds.), *Personality Change*. New York: Wiley.

GENDLIN, EUGENE (1981), *Focusing*. New York: Bantam Books.

GENDLIN, BEEBE, CASSENS, KLEIN, and OBERLANDER (1968), 'Focusing ability in psychotherapy, personality and creativity', *Research in Psychotherapy*, Vol. III, ed. J. Shlien. Washington, DC: American Psychological Association.

LEIJSSEN, MIA (1990), 'On focusing and the necessary conditions of therapeutic personality change', in G. Lietaer, J. Rombauts, and R. Van Balen (eds.), *Client-Centered and Experiential Psychotherapy in the Nineties*. Leuven, Belgium: Leuven University Press.

SIEMS, MARTIN (1986), *Dein Körper weiss die Antwort*. Hamburg: Rowohlt.

# · 9 ·

# Person-Centred Family Therapy

## NED L. GAYLIN

### INTRODUCTION

I began my career as a child therapist, and the vast majority of my professional life has been spent working with children and their families. Early on I learned that a family approach was the most efficacious means of working with troubled children. Working directly within the intimate interpersonal family context maximized the child's potential to experience positive and lasting change. I later found this to be true in psychotherapy with adults as well. As a result I have continued to be discomfited by the change of nomenclature from 'client-centred' to 'person-centred'. For me 'the client' is usually a couple or family group.

Nonetheless, I continue to feel most at home and congruent with the philosophy and tenets at the heart of the person-centred approach which respects and prizes the uniqueness of each individual person, each with his or her idiosyncratic process of growth. However, like George Herbert Mead (1934), it is my belief that there can be no person, no 'self', outside the interpersonal context. The human condition, by its very nature, is totally and completely interpersonal. Basic and paradigmatic to our interpersonal nature is the context in which that nature is shaped, the human family.

I had grown increasingly uncomfortable with the person-centred emphasis on 'independence' as a key concept in defining psychological well-being. Thus, in Chicago at the first meeting of the Association for the Development of the Person-Centered Approach (1986), I recall screwing up my courage and confronting Rogers on this point. Someone had asked him to define the 'healthy, or fully functioning person'. I remember being taken aback at the enormity of the question. However, Rogers did not flinch, and in his typical manner, went on to think aloud. I do not recall all of the characteristics he listed, because at the top of his list was the quality of 'independence'. I began to feel uncomfortable. Uncharacteristically for me, I interrupted him and suggested that the concept of an independent human being was antithetical to the human condition: indeed, *interdependence* defined our species. I expected an argument from Rogers. Instead, he paused, cocked his head, thoughtful for a moment, and agreed. That was it, just a simple agreement.

But I think I wanted, perhaps needed, an argument, or at least some dialogue on the matter. Despite Rogers' acquiescence, the person-centred philosophy really does stress the independent nature of the person.* Furthermore, I think that this emphasis on the individual hinders the actualizing of the person-centred approach into a more comprehensive theory of the human condition. Thus, until recently, I continued to use the older and, for me, more comfortable nomenclature of client-centred therapy whether my client was an individual, a couple, or a family. More recently, however, I began to use 'family-centred therapy' (Gaylin, 1989, 1990) to indicate the specific application of client-centred philosophy, theory, and methods to the practice of marriage and family therapy. Ironically, having just completed a paper (Gaylin, 1991b) on the development of the self in the family-centred context, I now realize that a person-centred family therapy could indeed be, not a contradiction in terms, but rather a more consonant form of family therapy than any of those commonly practised today.

---

* This underlying emphasis on individual independence as a quality of the fully functioning person may be seen in continued discussions on 'autonomy' and 'personal power' (e.g. Rogers, 1977; Natiello, 1987).

## THEORETICAL ISSUES

It well may be asked why it is necessary to belabour the theoretical and apparently abstract differences in the beliefs underlying our practice of psychotherapy. Put more pragmatically, how or why does theory affect the manner in which we conduct ourselves as psychotherapists? I believe the answer lies not so much in how theory changes our therapeutic techniques, but rather how theory affects our world-view of the process of change in our clients. This perspective, in turn, shapes our approach to our clients.

In the process of establishing itself as a distinct discipline, family therapy has, in the last twenty years, embraced various 'systems' models (see Nichols, 1984 and Auerswald, 1987). Despite their sometimes contradictory nature, all of the systems paradigms emphasize the family as a special unit, an entity far different from simply the sum of its individual parts. In fact, the one element common to virtually all the family systems models is the avoidance, in both theory and practice, of focusing on the intrapersonal dynamics of the individual family members.

On the other hand, the person-centred approach has traditionally emphasized the individual's internal dynamics. The individual's growth or self-actualization is the primary concern of the therapy hour. Despite the fact that this growth invariably has taken place in the context of a family of some sort, this context is of concern only as the client incidentally presents it to the therapist.

Although Rogers (1959, 1961, 1977) occasionally alluded to the family and the interaction among its members, such discussions were invariably brief and always couched in terms of the impact, either positive or negative, of familial interactions on the individual's actualizing tendency. Ironically, Rogers' psychology, not unlike that of Freud, is clearly oriented to the individual, the context being, at best, secondary.

Thus I must argue against any false theoretical dichotomy between individual and family therapy, a dichotomy in part created by the traditional individualism of the person-centred approach and by the intentional distinction made by those who saw family

183

therapy as a unique, iconoclastic, and revolutionary approach (e.g. Haley, 1963; Jackson, 1965; Minuchin, 1967). What I am arguing for is a person-centred therapy, which respects the individual, but which also considers and respects the context of that individual's development. This context, for virtually all of us, is the family.

The family unit is a living, organic whole that is never quite the same at any given moment in time. The family is continuously in flux because each person is composed of many self elements all of which are continuously experiencing change. These changes occur within the individual members through growth. In turn, changes of the self elements within the individual engender change – often subtle, sometimes dramatic – in the relationships among the individual's self elements and those of other family members.

The family may be seen as a kind of organic kaleidoscope composed of many selves, the elements of which are constantly changing in an interactive fluid environment. While the whole has an overall appearance which we all recognize, it is never quite the same from moment to moment. The interactive patterns are constantly changing due to the subtle shifts caused by both external and internal forces. Thus, there are at least three sources of change constantly affecting the family: (a) the intrapersonal dynamics of each of the individual family members which are fluid because of maturation and the accretion of experience; (b) the interpersonal interactions between and among members; and (c) the environmental forces, both natural and social, which bear upon the family from outside.

Person-centred theory enables our understanding of the individual's integrity, while family therapy augments understanding of the interpersonal nature of the human condition and the person's self-actualizing process. Therefore, I believe that a person-centred family therapy leads to a better understanding of couples and family groups, while reciprocally enhancing our understanding of individuals, since it is through interpersonal process that self-development occurs.

Yet, one of the glaring omissions in the person-centred literature is an understanding of how the self develops. Crucial to that understanding is the knowledge of how the individual is introduced to society. That introduction is accomplished by the family, the mediator between the individual and society. Furthermore, it is the family that initially swaddles the developing neonate in those conditions which Rogers (1957) deems necessary as well as sufficient for growth and change to take place, namely empathic unconditional positive regard. These conditions define love along with trust, and comprise the emotional bedrock of the family (Gaylin, 1991a). Indeed, the therapeutic relationship pales by any comparison with the actualizing power engendered by the family (Gaylin, 1990).

In the theory of person-centred therapy, the entire conceptualizing of the therapeutic relationship draws upon the analogue of the nurturance of the family during the early months and years of the individual's experience. Despite this parallel between the loving and trusting familial relationships and those same qualities found in the therapeutic relationship, person-centred theory virtually ignores the complexity of the developing person's relationships within the family.

Another oversight, not solely in the person-centred or humanistic literature, but in the behavioural sciences in general, is the neonate's contribution and participation in the relationship. As individuals we are each unique because of the distinctiveness of our genetic make-up. We are each conceived with genetically different constitutions which shape our temperaments (Thomas and Chess, 1977). In turn, each of our temperaments interacts with our equally unique complex familial environments to fashion our personalities. Conversely, from birth each of us has a special impact on our familial environments and its members (Bell, 1971). This complex interactional reciprocity and shaping begins at birth, perhaps at conception, and continues throughout our lives.

Although in theory the person-centred approach emphasizes the uniqueness of each individual, in practice this uniqueness tends to be disregarded because our theory suggests that all individuals should be treated in the same manner within the psychotherapy

185

session. What is often lost sight of is that each therapist–client relationship is idiosyncratic: each client/therapist pair interacts differently from every other pairing. Family therapy offers an opportunity to focus on the relationships between people as a central aspect of the healing process.

Except in disturbed families, there is a basic nurturance that is unconditional, and deeply empathic of the child's needs. Beyond this platform, however, the family, which by its very nature has no theoretical rule-book to guide it in its important task of engendering its new members, treats each person as distinctive. Thus, beginning with the first few months of life, each child in the family is dealt with differently.

However, as the child matures, parental love appears to grow conditional, often depending upon the child's behaviour and the parent's mood (Gaylin, 1991a). This is the process of socialization: learning to live in concert; learning that there are rights and privileges, but correspondingly, duties and obligations (Gaylin, 1980). Thus, the growing child's self emerges and is fashioned within the familial environment along with the child's sense of self-esteem. Individual differences and the corresponding 'goodness of fit' (Chess and Thomas, 1987) with the intimate environment of the family, will have enormous impact on how each of us feels about ourselves and the world around us throughout our lives.

Empathy from all indications is an innate human process and present in the infant from birth (Sagi and Hoffman, 1976). By means of empathy the very young person relates to others and the self emerges. This emergence of self begins first through the process of self-awareness, then through self-differentiation during the first year (Brunner, 1986); it is crystallized before the end of the second year of life (Mahler, Pine, and Bergman, 1975). Thus, through empathy, putting oneself in the place of the other, that sentience and true humanness develop.

Within the first two years, the child develops language. Nomenclatural understanding of intimate relationships in the environment defines the self of the child in context. This contextual or relational self becomes an amalgam of many *subselves* which the individual accretes throughout the life course.*

We start out as a child, utterly dependent upon our primary caretakers. The dependent child self is the first of many that will emerge from the beginnings of our awareness of self as an acting and interacting entity. Soon this self may be extended, depending upon family constellation, by a sibling self and we begin the lifelong process of defining ourselves by our interaction and relationship with others in our environment. Thus, we begin amassing a set of *subselves* that creates a *self-complex* (Gaylin, 1991b) by which we define ourselves.

The understanding of the *self-complex* and the subtle interactions of our various *subselves* within that *self-complex* is crucial to an understanding of psychological well-being. Our self-esteem at any given moment in time is affected by this ever-changing constellation of selves, which is idiosyncratic to each of us, and is dependent upon history, internal constitutional environment, and the external environmental context in which we are operating. Thus, our internal states, such as hunger and fatigue, may affect our self-evaluations, as will external forces such as the weather, interpersonal threat, and so on. Furthermore, this self-evaluation is complicated by changes regarding which of our many *subselves* we deem pre-eminent at any given moment in time. For example, when I am at home, my spousal or parental *subself* may be pre-eminent; while at the university, the teacher or collegial *subself* may take precedence as the locus of my evaluation of self. These evaluations are continuously fluid, changing with time and environment, as well as with biological state and mood.†

The question that arises is how the self-complex is managed,

---

* Throughout this discussion the use of the word 'role' is intentionally avoided as counterproductive to the understanding of the development of the complex self (see Gaylin, 1991b).

† These ideas are not new, nor unique to the person-centred approach. Indeed, they form the antecedents to the person-centred thinking of Rogers. They draw upon William James' 'hierarchy of selves' (1890), G. H. Mead's 'interactive self' (1934) and H. S. Sullivan's development of self through communication (1953).

how we maintain some sense of self-integrity, wholeness, or self-identity. It is this question that has intrigued the earliest philosophers and is the engine that continues to drive psychological theorists. The human condition is unique because of our memory of the past and our ability to transcend our immediate past through both oral and written history. This trans-temporal awareness is, undoubtedly, intimately related to at least two features of our biological uniqueness: (a) our highly developed cortical functioning and (b) our long neonatal dependence (Gaylin, 1985, 1991a).

James (1890) speaks of our awareness of self and our sense of its continuity through time as a 'stream of consciousness' that keeps our selves intact, flowing from one experience to another. For this sense of self-continuity, I prefer a slightly less fluid metaphor, that of a weaving or tapestry, the warp threads of which are shaped by our biological constitutions, our genetic heritage, and laid out by our earliest interpersonal experience within our families. This warp forms the foundation of our fabric, with subsequent experience serving as the weft. Thus, our selfhood is like a continuous fabric which maintains integrity over time despite change in texture, colour, and design.

The person-centred approach is an interesting alloy of self and experiential postulates. Basically, to review what has been stated earlier, the *self-complex* is composed of many *subselves* which evolve and constantly are reshaped by interpersonal experiences. The process of psychotherapy is one more of those experiences, but one that focuses on the process of experiencing itself. In a safe interpersonal environment, the client proactively examines and re-experiences aspects of the self complex.

Psychotherapy is modern science's analogue for other enriching interpersonal experiences, such as loving familial relationships, intimate friendships, and communion with God, all of which serve to heal and enhance the person. Such healing relationships and experiences were reported in both sacred and secular literature long before the advent of psychotherapy. These experiences continue to be a source of solace for the vast majority of humankind. Perhaps it is time for psychotherapy to learn from these relationships and incorporate their restorative qualities into our theory and practice.

The premiss of individual psychotherapy has been that we can mitigate emotional suffering by examining our life experience with a therapist. How much more efficacious might the therapeutic endeavour be if, with a therapist, we explored these experiences with people who have been a part of our emotional development and continue to share our most intimate life space.

## FROM THEORY TO PRACTICE

Based on the theoretical premises stated above I choose to do person-centred therapy in the context of a marriage or a family. When individuals call me for therapy, I often will suggest that they bring their spouse or other significant family members with them to at least our first session, if the individuals feel comfortable in so doing. If an interpersonal problem exists and has precipitated the call, I frequently suggest that the caller bring the individual with whom they are experiencing difficulties. Of course sometimes this is neither desirable nor realistic: if one is experiencing difficulties with one's boss, it might be neither easy nor desirable to take the boss in to see one's therapist. Sometimes, if one is trying to divorce, leave, or disengage from a relationship, and is having difficulty doing so, the last thing one might want is to have that person in the room. On the other hand, had we a different way of looking at the power of the therapeutic process, it might be exactly the thing to do. Since virtually all therapy deals with issues of interpersonal relationships, the inclusion of others should be looked upon not as unusual and odd, but usual and natural.

To have people who are important to my client present in therapy allows me, in part, to make myself familiar to those persons. But that is the least of why that presence is important. Almost immediately, even my most sceptical clients discover the profound usefulness of having along a significant person, someone to turn to for validation of perceptions and experiential details which facilitate more readily the client's examination of his or herself in the life context. From here the therapeutic process continues naturally.

It is interesting to note that the person-centred approach has used relationship milieu techniques in more traditional settings, specifically with groups (see Bebout, 1974, and Beck, 1974) for some time. On the other hand, I am puzzled that so few of my person-centred colleagues venture into similar work with couples and families. In part, I believe that spending part of one's therapy hours in work with families is not only consonant with the person-centred approach, but greatly enhances the therapist's ability to understand human problems, and thereby facilitate more successful work with those clients whose family members may not be available.

Although the morphology of the family-centred hour may appear vastly different from that of an individual client-centred hour, the work of the therapist is often virtually the same. Commonly the person-centred family therapist starts out by responding in a manner not unlike that of an individual client-centred therapist, listening to a family member, and empathically reflecting that member's message.

Because family therapy generally deals with the conflict and incongruities between and among family members, usually other family members will counter with their perceptions of the given situation, and the therapist then may empathically respond to each family member in turn.

A subtle but palpable difference between the behaviour of the family therapist and that of the individual therapist is that the family therapist may, at times, need to mediate when conflicts become heated. That is, there is a tendency for individual members to become agitated over stated and perceived discrepancies that may prevail. In dismay and disbelief, one or more members may attempt to interrupt another family member engaged in an elucidation of his or her perceptions. In such circumstances the therapist may have to manage the session so that all family members are reassured that each will be heard.

The therapist, once having empathically responded to everyone's position, continues by relating an understanding of each person's internal frame of reference. Sometimes this is sufficient, but sometimes it is helpful for the therapist to summarize the shared and conflicted meanings within the family unit.

Because of their own individual frames of reference, it is sometimes difficult for some family members to comprehend another member's perceptions, and feelings. Consequently, it is not uncommon, particularly during early family therapy sessions, for members to make attributions regarding other members' thoughts, attitudes, and feelings. The following fictitious scenario with Ruth, a teenager, and her parents is representative of such a situation.

Ruth, to her parents: 'You never understand how I feel about such and such.' The family therapist can rechannel such attributions by reflecting them, and might say: 'When you tell Mom and Dad about your feelings about such and such it seems to you they never understand you.' In return one of the parents may respond with something like: 'We want to understand, but every time we try and talk to you about it, you get angry and walk away.' Then the therapist might respond to the parents: 'When you try and understand what Ruth is troubled about, you feel she doesn't hear your questions or your concern.'

At a moment like this the therapist is in the position of reflecting what I refer to as the *interspace* between and among the family members, and might comment accordingly: 'Whenever you try to talk about such and such there seems to be some kind of wall between you.' In this manner the individuals have been heard and the problem couched in such a manner that no one is blamed or held responsible for the conflict but, rather, the situation is described and the conflict exposed allowing for examination in a less emotionally debilitating manner.

Despite their apparent simplicity, reflecting each person's stance and the interpersonal interspaces often results in the reduction of attribution and blame-laying. Thus, detailed, personally experiential recounting of highly charged conflict-laden family interactions which the family has previously found counterproductive often promotes increased understanding and creative problem solving on the part of the family and its members.

191

Unlike other family therapy modalities, the family-centred therapist does not attempt to resolve the problem, but, rather, creates the facilitative and engendering atmosphere in which the family may reconceptualize its problems, concerns, and goals. In this manner, the family's actualizing tendency (Gaylin, 1990) can be disencumbered and psychotherapeutic change can take place.

On the other hand, working with families, particularly families in which there are young children, entails certain complexities with which the client-centred therapist working exclusively with individuals is rarely, if ever, confronted. Such complications concern the normative development of children. Parents worried that their children are not walking or talking by the age of two years may indeed have children with pragmatic developmental problems. The presence of constitutional dysfunctions in children does not deny the reality, nor mitigate the necessity of dealing with the emotional anguish and concern that invariably accompany such developmental difficulties. However, it would be both dangerous and professionally derelict to deal with the latter without dealing with the former. Conversely, there are occasions when parental expectations of a child may be inappropriately high *vis-à-vis* the child's developmental readiness, thereby creating both intrapersonal and interpersonal incongruence.

Thus, therapists working with the families of young children should have a basic knowledge of child development including appropriate intervention options when delays are apparent or disorders become manifest. Although I believe it is important for a family therapist to be comfortable and able to work in a child guidance mode, it may be sufficient for some therapists to know when it is necessary to make a referral. Note that there is a distinction being made between family therapy and child guidance. Although some therapists may do both within the context of a family therapy hour, I consider it essential to recognize and separate the two processes, and know when to do which, and why. Such recognition is crucial to the therapist's own congruence and integrity as a person-centred family therapist.

Appreciation of the family is an organic as well as cultural whole faces the person-centred family therapist with the need for additional awareness. There is a natural hierarchy within all families: the younger generation accords respect to their parents by dint of their ages and their parental roles. Although some cultures may tend to de-emphasize this hierarchy, it is nonetheless a feature of all families in all cultures. In families with teenage children, the therapist's empathic stance towards a teenager attempting to come to grips with struggles of independence may too easily be misinterpreted by a parent as the therapist's approbation and support of the child's disrespectful position towards the parents.

Out of recognition and respect for the responsibility and authority of the parents, I invariably ask them to come alone for the first session in order to: (a) give them an opportunity to know me and establish a relationship; (b) listen to their perceptions of the problem(s); and (c) allow me to explain how, on occasion, my attention and empathy may appear more focused on their child. I have never had a parent misunderstand my position during the therapy hour when I have contracted in this manner. On the other hand, severe misunderstandings have been created on those exceptional occasions when I have not followed this procedure. Once the initial contracting stage has been accomplished, I am comfortably guided by the family's expressed needs regarding which family members should attend the therapy hour.

This introductory approach to the family is at odds with many family therapy modalities which advocate seeing the entire family from the outset. My approach also runs counter to that of some other person-centred family therapists (e.g. Levant, 1984, and Thayer, 1982) who see the family as the sole decider of who is to attend sessions and when. However, I consider these opening decisions on my part well within the client-centred framework: in much the same way an individual client-centred therapist sets the length of the hour, the time and spacing of the visits, etc. to meet the mutual needs of both client and therapist.

Another example of an extension of client-centred thinking is a particular method that I came upon through a confluence of the experiences of teaching family studies while working clinically with individuals, couples, and families. For want of a better term, I have temporarily called the method *ghosting*.*

Basically *ghosting* is a means of empathizing with an absent member. I accidentally stumbled upon this method when teaching an introductory course on marriage and family therapy to graduate students. Not infrequently, after class, individual participants would come to my office to discuss a problem that they were having with a spouse or parent. As they related some troublesome incident or problem that they were having in this relationship, they would ask my advice about what to do. After deferring and suggesting that they seek professional counselling, I would try to be empathic with the student and his or her anguish in the interpersonal situation that they had just related. I then would add comments such as, 'You know, if you had said such and such to me, I might have felt hurt, or upset, although I might not have been able to tell you so at the time.' Frequently, I would hear later from these students that they had related my statement back to the person with whom they had been having difficulty. The person would agree that my description of my probable feelings given the same circumstances closely matched their feelings. The student would often go on to note that a meaningful conversation ensued which subsequently helped resolve the difficulty.

The empathic stance with an absent member has often been more meaningful and powerful in marital or family therapy when, on occasion, I have been asked to see one member of the family and the other member(s) could not be present. It should be noted that seeing a family member without the rest of the family or a partner without the spouse is a practice I avoid, particularly in the beginning of therapy (except in some parent–child therapy, as previously noted). However, on occasion when a spouse has had to be out of town, and has supported such an arrangement, I have agreed to see the remaining partner alone.

* Although to some this method may appear similar to the 'empty chair' and 'doubling' techniques used in psychodrama (Moreno, 1947), I prefer not to think of this way of working as simply another technique but, rather, an indigenous outgrowth of the empathic stance.

Having worked with the absent member, and therefore having had an ongoing relationship with that member, I have been able to adopt an empathic position with him or her. As a consequence, I have been free to say something in response to the present client such as, 'You know, I think I understand how you feel about such and such' (being more empathically specific), 'and I wonder if John were here, whether or not he might see things differently, more like this' (and have proceeded to offer a hypothetical comment about John's possible feelings). Thus, I have *ghosted* the absent member.

To my *ghosting* comments the partner present has often cocked his or her head, literally or figuratively, and processed this new data in a manner which, reportedly, has provided new insights into the situation. Furthermore, the partner who was present would invariably report the episode to the absent member. This, in turn, would have at least two beneficial results: first, a continued clarifying exchange between the partners; and second, a building of trust with me insofar as I was able to continue to respond empathically to both members, even when one was absent.

I would like to re-emphasize that I do not look upon *ghosting* simply as a technique, but rather as a natural extension of the person-centred approach of employing empathy and prizing stances within the therapeutic relationship. Thus, practising person-centred family therapy has enabled my ability to more clearly identify the interpersonal elements which I believe are integral to all clients' psychological incongruence.

Perhaps, more importantly, *ghosting* clarifies the implications and ramifications of person-centred family therapy and its potential power. Thus, being aware of the *subselves* within the *self-complex*, one is cognizant of the fact that the child self in all of us exists, ready to be called upon should the appropriate experiential conditions prevail. For example, although my parents, through whom I originally defined myself as a child, are no longer alive, when I think of them I think of myself as their child. Death may end active involvement with a significant person in our lives, but it does not end the relationship.

Thus, when working with families, the therapist may observe

the empathic resonance of family members for one another as the empathic process between the therapist and a given family member takes place. One can see, as the therapy unfolds, how this resonance continues to infuse the family process over time, even as the actualizing tendency of the family as a whole (Gaylin, 1990) begins to be mobilized.

I learned the power of this kind of resonance personally, through an incident that occurred about a generation ago. My father had died when I was a young man, married, yet without children. My father was a wonderful and gentle man but, as many others of his generation of Polish-Russian immigrants, rather stern and authoritative. He died, just as I was beginning to appreciate him as a person, not simply a loving authority figure. We never really had an opportunity to become friends.

About ten years after my father's death, an incident occurred when our son, the youngest of our four children, was about four years old. It should be noted that he was relationally in the identical position to me as I to my father (i.e. I was the youngest of three and my son the youngest of four; I had been born when my father was in early middle age, so was my son). I was minding the children while my wife was running errands, and Daniel, the most spirited of our children, was playing near me as I was doing some work at my desk.

Out of the corner of my eye – I had learned to look out of the corner of my eye when Daniel was particularly quiet – I noticed that he had somehow managed to pull the uppermost file drawer out of a very heavy old oak four-drawer filing cabinet and had begun swinging on it. The cabinet began to lean and topple, and would almost immediately and inevitably fall squarely on Daniel. I, terrified, leaped out of my chair just in time to grab him and slam the drawer shut before the cabinet could fall. Adrenalized and shaking, my fear converted to anger now that the catastrophe had been avoided, I began shouting at my four-year-old son, who stood in front of me, not quite comprehending all that had transpired in those frightening seconds.

Furious, I excoriated him. As I felt the ugly words tumble from my mouth, I saw tears well up in Daniel's eyes. The image triggered a memory trace, never before retrieved. At that instant two other people, almost literally in my mind's eye, joined us. These apparitions were myself at Daniel's age, who now stood next to him, and my father, at my age, who stood just to the right, and behind me.

As I saw my words hit their mark, I saw, and felt, the four-year-old me crying alongside my tearful son. I knew exactly what my son was experiencing, and a part of me wanted to grab him and hug him and tell him how much I loved him, and explain that I was angry at him because I was so frightened for both of us. But I could neither say these things nor stop the abusive words being hurled at him from my mouth. I felt tears welling up in my own eyes and, never looking behind me to my right for fear my father would disappear if I did so, I felt myself wanting to embrace my father and tell him that now I finally understood.

That moment was an experiential fulcrum in my life, as I realized that my many *subselves* maintained themselves in my stream of consciousness; that the many aspects of me continued to exist within me as I related to significant others in my life space, the living and the dead. It has called itself up in my memory many times in individual therapy, but far more so in family therapy sessions as I see children and their parents struggling to understand each other, as I empathize with their struggle and attempt to help them in the process. It is part of what makes me a person-centred family therapist.*

REFERENCES

AUERSWALD, E. H. (1987), 'Epistemological confusion in family therapy research', *Family Process*, 26, September, 317–30.
BEBOUT, J. (1974), 'It takes one to know one: Existential-Rogerian

---

* For want of a better label, I have called this experience *intergenerational echoing*.

concepts in encounter groups', in L. N. Rice and D. Wexler (eds.), *Innovations in Client-Centered Therapy*. New York: John Wiley and Sons.

BECK, A. P. (1974), 'Phases in the development of structure in therapy and encounter groups', in L. N. Rice and D. Wexler (eds.), *Innovations in Client-Centered Therapy*. New York: John Wiley and Sons.

BELL, R. Q. (1971), 'Stimulus control of parent or caretaker behavior by offspring', *Developmental Psychology*, 4, 63–72.

BRUNNER, J. (1986), *Actual Minds, Possible Worlds*. Cambridge: Harvard University Press.

CHESS, S., and THOMAS, A. (1987), *Know Your Child*. New York: Basic Books.

GAYLIN, N. L. (1980), 'Rediscovering the family', in N. Stinett, B. Chesser, J. Defrain, and B. Knaub (eds.), *Family Strengths: positive models for family life*. Lincoln, Neb.: University of Nebraska Press.

GAYLIN, N. L. (1985), 'Marriage: the civilizing of sexuality', in M. Farber (ed.), *Human Sexuality: psychosocial aspects of disease*. New York: Macmillan and Co.

GAYLIN, N. L. (1989), 'The necessary and sufficient conditions for change: individual versus family therapy', *Person-Centered Review*, 4, 263–69.

GAYLIN, N. L. (1990), 'Family-centered therapy', in G. Lietaer, J. Rombauts, and R. Van Balen (eds.), *Client-Centered and Experiential Psychotherapy in the Nineties*. Leuven, Belgium: Leuven University Press.

GAYLIN, N. L. (1991a), 'An intergenerational perspective of marriage: love and trust in cultural context', in S. Pfiefer and M. Sussman (eds.), *Families: intergenerational and generational connections*. New York: Haworth Press.

GAYLIN, N. L. (1991b), 'Family-centered theory: the client-centered relationship in developmental context.' Paper presented at the Second International Conference on Client-Centred and Experiential Psychotherapy, University of Stirling, Scotland.

HALEY, J. (1963), *Strategies of Psychotherapy*. New York: Grune and Stratton.

JACKSON, D. D. (1965), 'Family rules: marital quid pro quo', *Archives of General Psychiatry*. 1, 618–21.

JAMES, W. (1890), *The Principles of Psychology*. New York: Holt.

LEVANT, R. (1984), 'From person to system: two perspectives', in R. Levant and J. Shlien (eds.), *Client-Centered Therapy and the Person-Centered Approach: new directions in theory, research, and practice*. New York: Prager.

MAHLER, M. S., PINE, F., and BERGMAN, A. (1975), *The Psychological Birth of the Infant*. New York: Basic Books.

MEAD, G. H. (1934), *Mind, Self, and Society*. Chicago: University of Chicago Press.

MINUCHIN, S. (1964), *Families and Family Therapy*. Cambridge, Mass: Harvard University Press.

MORENO, J. L. (1947), *The Theater of Spontaneity: an introduction to psychodrama*. New York: Beacon House.

NATIELLO, P. (1987), 'The person-centered approach: from theory to practice', *Person-Centered Review*, 2, 203–16.

NICHOLS, M. (1984), *Family Therapy: concepts and methods*. New York: Gardner Press.

ROGERS, C. R. (1959), 'A theory of therapy, personality and inter-personal relationships as developed in the client-centered framework', in S. Koch (ed.), *Psychology: a study of a science, Vol. III. Formulations of the person and the social context*. New York: McGraw Hill.

ROGERS, C. R. (1961), *On Becoming a Person*. Boston: Houghton Mifflin.

ROGERS, C. R. (1977), *Carl Rogers on Personal Power*. New York: Dell.

SAGI, A., and HOFFMAN, M. L. (1976), 'Empathic distress in the newborn', *Developmental Psychology*, 12, 175–76.

SULLIVAN, H. S. (1953), *The Interpersonal Theory of Psychiatry*. New York: W. W. Norton.

THAYER, L. (1982), 'A person-centered approach to family therapy', in A. M. Horne and M. M. Ohlsen (eds.), *Family Counseling and Therapy*. Itasca, Ill: F. E. Peacock.

THOMAS, A., and CHESS, S. (1977), *Temperament and Development*. New York: Brunner/Mazel.

# · 10 ·

# Encounter Group Experiences of Black and White South Africans in Exile

## E. SALEY AND LEN HOLDSTOCK

'Goodbye, small farmhouse and my native country. I leave you as a young man leaves his mother: he knows it is time for him to leave her, and he knows, too, he can never leave her completely, even though he wants to.'

Herman Hesse, *Farmhouse* (1920)

'There is no greater sorrow than the loss of one's fatherland.'

Euripides, 431 BC (in *Amnesty International*, 1987)

Civil wars and the persecution of dissidents are a feature of our history as old as humankind. Indeed, the chronicle of our species from its first page recounts tragic tales of oppression and flight from persecution. This legacy has persisted over time and much of our present world still faces the problems of large numbers of exiles who are tragically 'caught between the violence at home and the loss of identity in a strange and distant land' (Stein, 1986).

Exiles are forced to leave home or, to use Kunz's (1973) term, are 'pushed' out because it is the only alternative to the violence and persecution in their own native lands. Theirs is an involuntary departure necessitated by reasons of political or ideological belief and self-preservation. Thus, an exile's journey is started not in anticipation of a better life elsewhere, but is compelled by personal conviction and the fear of persecution. For them the option of returning home is ruled out as long as the reasons that made them leave persist. Herein lies the essential difference between exiles and other migrants: for the exile, departure is imposed and return impossible.

The predicament that an exile is confronted with on arriving in the country of asylum is as complex as it is compelling. He or she is faced with a profound loss of family, culture, identity and status. Exiles suddenly find themselves virtual 'islands in a strange and often hostile sea' (Mutiso, 1979). Whereas previously they may have had social and political status as leaders, intellectuals and activists within their own communities, they suddenly become non-entities among people vastly different from themselves.

This sense of alienation often causes the exile to become depressed, frustrated, bitter and resentful toward the new country and its people. In trying to deal with this crushing sense of isolation, an exile often comes to deny the present by 'clinging to the familiar and changing no more than necessary' (Scudder and Colson, 1982), thereby becoming a prisoner of a self-idealizing past and a future characterized by the hope of ultimately returning home. As the exiled South African journalist Malan (1990) eloquently puts it, 'I yearned to sit again with anguished socialists over mugs of tea in cold slum kitchens, talking politics, for even then, at our lowest and most miserable, life was a larger stage and you were on it, playing your allotted part. I often wished I'd stayed at home, or that I could go back, but I couldn't; I might have been jailed as a draft evader' (p. 76). Paradoxically, in many cases the greater the impossibility of returning home the more cherished the illusion of returning becomes.

This fixation on the past-identity and rejection of the present functions like a two-edged sword. If left uncontrolled it can become destructive and pathological. However, if nurtured and channelled correctly it becomes a vital stimulus for self-discovery and growth. Herein lies the challenge to mental health workers dealing with exiles.

In the South African exile community in Amsterdam a great deal of unhappiness and polarization between black and white members was evident. Although person-centred therapy has not been applied to work done with exiles, the known effectiveness of person-centred encounter groups in facilitating personal growth (Rogers, 1970; Sanford, 1984), suggested itself as a method to be used in facilitating the psychological adjustments of South African exiles in The Netherlands.

## PROCEDURE

The encounter group was started under the auspices of the Amsterdam-based South African Community and Culture Centre (SACCC) in May 1988 and lasted until June 1990. The encounter group was initially focused at resolving the inter-racial conflicts within the exiled community of South Africans living in The Netherlands. Participation was invited through an announcement in the SACCC newsletter that reached approximately three hundred exiles all over The Netherlands. The announced purpose of the encounter group was 'to provide interested black and white South African exiles with the opportunity to encounter each other on a person-to-person level within an honest and non-coercive environment'. The group met once a week for two hours at a time.

The first meeting was attended by twenty persons but in subsequent sessions participation dropped to an average of twelve members per session. People were allowed to join and leave at any time. In total about thirty people attended. Some participated in only one or two sessions. Eight members remained in the group throughout its duration.

In the beginning the group was representative (although not proportionally) of the four official (as prescribed by the South African regime) racial denominations in South Africa. However, there were only two women and fewer black than white participants. All the white participants were from English-speaking backgrounds.

All the group participants were resident in The Netherlands. Except for two white participants, the others had official status as asylum seekers which entitled them to such benefits as social security, legal employment, health benefits and the possibility of Dutch nationality after five years in the country. The length of time that members had spent in exile varied, the longest being fourteen and the most recent just over one year.

The youngest member was nineteen and the eldest was fifty old. There was a diversity of occupations and educational levels represented within the group. There were authors, actors, musicians, poets, playwrights, artists, teachers, students, a professional story-teller, a technician, a builder, a clerk and a model. Of the eight permanent participants, four were university graduates and the rest had varying levels of schooling.

Generally all the white male members left South Africa as conscientious objectors, either resisting compulsory conscription or deserting from the South African army. The black members were either escaping the violence or avoiding detention. Because the South African community in The Netherlands is relatively small, most of the group members were known to each other before the encounter group began.

During the first five months the use of a tape recorder was not allowed by the group because of the 'spy-phobia' prevalent among most political exiles. Coincidentally, the group meetings occurred before and during the period when major political changes took place in South Africa. Consequently, the group experience can be divided into the periods before and after political change.

## RESULTS

At the beginning, the group discussions centred around black–white relationships within the community in Amsterdam. Despite the fact that the group members were all against the policies of the South African government, their relationships were still polarized in terms of skin colour. The polarization was especially evident in the unwitting use of language and other forms of expression with racist connotations by some white members. Terms such as 'kaffir-beer', 'garden-boy' and 'natives' have become so much part and parcel of the vocabulary of white South Africans, that even 'politically enlightened' persons were unaware of the racist overtones of these terms. The following extract serves as an example of such language use.

> I remember being scared. There was this open veld behind our house where these natives used to gather and drink their kaffir-beer and dance and make a noise. One night my parents were not home and they were coming into our yard. I remember sitting there with the doors locked and rifle in hand protecting my younger sisters and brother. We were children and we were scared of them.

Even though the offending language referred to the past and to usage by people other than the group member, as indicated in the following extract, it still tended to polarize group relationships and at times evoked angry responses.

> In my home the black gardener being referred to as the 'garden boy' was in a way a legacy from the British colonial days. Calling an adult a 'boy' or 'girl' was a way of 'de-sexing' him or her. It helped to ease our fear of them. By referring to them as children, they became less of a threat.

It was felt that such language showed 'insensitivity to black members'. One black member remarked that he did not leave South Africa and come to Europe to find that even here he had to educate the white man. In this instance the black member withdrew from the group.

In another incident it was the nature of the paintings of a white member which evoked conflict.

> S.: Al's paintings for Soweto Day made me realize that even though we are all 'the converted' here, we still see 'the other side' in a way that fits our own perceptions. Particularly the one [painting] with the black woman dancing in a jungle setting seemed to be the ideal white stereotype of blacks. M. was furious because he felt insulted and the musicians were complaining that

some of the sketches of torture were too upsetting. That was the reason why we asked you to take them off even though some people accused us of censorship.

Al: I did not mean to offend anyone. I just tried to convey the truth of what I believed and when I heard of the goings on I withdrew. I'm sorry if my work came across as insensitive but that has been my isolation in exile. Soweto Day was my opportunity to come out and display the things inside. I am sorry that it caused so much trouble.

In the early sessions, the black participants recounted stories about growing up in black townships and how they perceived 'the other side'. The following examples indicate the nature of these statements:

My mother was a servant in a white house and she only came home on a Friday. We children looked forward to her coming because she always brought food from her white boss's house. So once a week we ate well . . . my grandmother always said that the food was a curse and I could never understand this. Now I understand.

Another black member said that he sometimes went with his mother to her work and that the people there were very good to him. They gave him clothes and toys because they had a son about his age. 'He was my friend, I learned to swim in their swimming pool, but I always felt very sad whenever I got things from him because I never had anything that I could give him in return.' About the white friend, he said that he saw him one day in town, dressed in army clothes. 'We looked at one another and passed one another without saying a word.'

White members reciprocated with anecdotes that described mostly the negative aspects of their upbringing. One said that politics and religion were taboo in his home and that he, too, became part of 'that collective conspiracy of silence'. Another said that he recalled the time when the Immorality Act was 'big'. He used to spy on his neighbour to see if he was not sneaking a black woman into his house. 'For me as a child I saw it as my duty to phone the police if that man took a black woman into his house . . . I have always wanted to make my parents proud by one day becoming a paratrooper. These were the values I was brought up with.'

The recollections of the white group members of black–white interactions in South Africa were generally of an employee-employer relationship. White members frequently mentioned their black maids in South Africa who were fondly referred to as 'black mother' or 'surrogate mother'. 'I still write to my black mother and when I can, I send money. I hope I can see her again one day.' In reply to the statement by a white member that he had two mothers, the one during the day and the one at night, and that he loved them both, a black member responded with the following telling statement: 'I gave up mine so that you could have two.'

In instances of direct confrontation, the group usually worked together in defusing serious conflicts. A much-used strategy was to shift the blame on to the system by constantly reaffirming that 'we are all victims of apartheid'.

Generally the sessions started with someone reporting a significant news item relating to South Africa. This was followed by a brief discussion. This feature persisted and became something of a group tradition.

After about five months, there was a marked change in the frequency and level of self-disclosure in the group. The white members increasingly expressed the need 'to confess the paradoxes' in their lives. The group became an opportunity 'to forgive yourself for past actions'. In the words of one group member, 'We are all victims of victims in South Africa!' 'Even love, the need for warmth, became corrupted in that system,' another said.

One of the predominant themes among white members was the 'turning point' or the 'moment of realization' when the decision to leave South Africa was made. In the words of one member:

It was a Saturday night and I was with some of my buddies at a roadhouse. Suddenly, out of the night a white man came running to us, his head was bleeding and all he had to say was that he was attacked by a black. That was it, we never ask who is right or wrong, the thing was that a black attacked a white man. We found the black guy in a yard, he was with his girlfriend in the servant's room. He ran and we chased and cornered him, there were six of us and we stood in a circle around him. He was being hit from all sides but he refused to fall. It became a challenge for us to see who would be able to drop him. It was at that moment, seeing that man who refused to fall that . . . I saw myself. It was something that I would do . . . that was me. A cop showed up and he said he was going to show us how to make this . . . 'kaffir' fall. He put handcuffs on the man and pressed . . . with the pain, the man screamed and sank to his knees. It was at that moment that something broke inside of me. It was like a sound, a crack. That was it, I was never going to be the same again. That was my moment of truth. I knew that I could never be part of that life again.

For other white members the decision to go into exile occurred while they were undergoing their compulsory conscription in the army. One person said that as a homosexual in the South African army, he was treated like a 'queer'.

They did not know what to do with me. They put me in with the medics. It was not easy for me . . . We were doing drills and it was staged in a way that the shooting range was situated near the fence. On the other side of the fence was the black township. We had to march up and down along the fence. There were these people from the townships looking at us and that's when it came to me. What were we doing with all this marching, learning to shoot and carrying out manoeuvres? It was rehearsing for murder. That's what we were doing in front of all those people, rehearsing for their murder.

For another group member the moment of truth occurred after he had been called up for commando duty in Alexandria township.

208

We had to back up the police in minding a road-block. For me this was a first trip to the township . . . and in the early morning we were dismissed. As I was leaving, a friend asked me to come home with him. He said that he had a surprise for me. So we went off to his place and he had these two beautiful black ladies staying with him. It was then that it struck me, just a few hours before I could have been responsible for killing their brothers or sisters and here I was planning to make love to one of them. This schizophrenia, this utter contradiction made me decide to get out.

As is apparent from the above extracts and also from the following interaction among group members the depth of self-disclosure increased in time:

G. (white): I was in a reformatory. It was a very difficult time for me because I was very lonely. I remember I used to walk the streets and find a black girl who was probably just as lonely as me. She would take me to her room and I would give her fifty cents . . . and she would be some warmth for me in my loneliness. And then I would come back to the dormitory and try and wash myself clean of everything. I would be in the shower for an hour washing the memory of her black body from me. This kept on repeating itself with maids in my mother's house. It was probably my rebellion against my mother, against my society . . . my pattern of breaking taboos in that way.

I.K. (white): I have also done plenty in that way. Most white boys have done that, taking black girls sexually happened all the time. And to be honest, for me at that age it was a matter of where I could get it and getting a black girl was easier. It was not because I was lonely.

Self-disclosure was observed mostly among the white members. The main contribution of black members at this stage was their continuing presence in the group. This presence implied 'acceptance' and in a way facilitated the 'mourning of the past'. The group interactions during this phase were past oriented. There was a clear separation between South Africa the motherland and South Africa the apartheid state. Whereas the motherland was idealized by all members, the state was denounced as the reason for all the unhappiness. Then the political change was heralded in by President de Klerk in his dramatic speech to Parliament (2 February 1990). In this speech he announced the release of Nelson Mandela and the unbanning of banned political organizations. This had a profound influence on the group.

The group discussions following de Klerk's speech became increasingly *future* oriented. 'Going home' became the central focus of the group discussions. For some members the thought of returning was idealized. One person said that he would like to live in a rondavel in the countryside, another that he would like to live on the farm of a friend where fresh water came out of a hill. Others were more cautious. 'It would be better to wait and see, and not let our expectations rise too high.' Some group members believed that 'being able to return is one thing, but apartheid is not yet abolished completely, and as long as it persists there can be no going back'. Others wanted to return so that they could 'contribute to the process of change in South Africa'.

The group discussion became more political in nature. As members spent more time debating their various political positions, the focus shifted from black–white differences towards differences between radical and moderate voices in the group. The new emphasis on politics and the future in South Africa caused somewhat of a rift in the cohesiveness which had developed in the group. The following are some examples of different political opinions that were expressed by the group members:

The ANC is going into negotiations with the government and I fear that what will happen is that we will end up with a reformed kind of apartheid. (White member.)

There can be no change until there is a redistribution of wealth. (White member.)

This scramble to get back, I am reminded of lemmings, it starts with one and the rest follow ... I am going to wait. I have read what the ANC wrote about the future of South Africa and I am not optimistic. (White member.)

My fear is the manipulation and the interest of the money houses here in Europe. It's going so fast that I believe that the magic and dignity of the old tribal ways are being betrayed. (White member.)

In ex-Rhodesia after independence they had national reconciliation. If that were to happen to South Africa, I would not feel satisfied. We have been fighting to establish a new society but in this time so much has been done wrong. I would not be satisfied until all those people are tried. (White member.)

I was reading an article in which they asked black people what they thought about apartheid going. In this article, they said that 40 per cent of the black rural population prefer to be ruled by a white president instead of a black one. (Black member.)

Members of the South African Youth Congress are working with the youth from the Afrikaner Broederbond ... they share common platforms. They differ on the issue of the armed struggle only but they decided not to make it an issue and to hold on to the common thing between them which is to fight apartheid. So there is more understanding at home. I think it should also happen here. (Black member.)

For many group members, the family at home became the central reason for either staying or returning. White group members were faced with the fact that by returning they would be confronted by the bigotry in their families. The following is an extreme example of such a dilemma:

I would not feel satisfied unless my father was tried ... he has a lot to answer for. I know him and I don't think that he will ever stop believing in his heart that what they are doing is right.

He is a member of the AWB [Afrikaner Weerstands Beweging] and probably one of the most extreme. Before 1985–1986, before everything started, he was reasonable. He did not get involved in politics and then all of a sudden he got involved with the police. He had many schemes going and with the help of his police friends he could make more money. I tried to appeal to him but he made me read all the AWB propaganda. If I opposed him on a political level, he called me a communist. If I opposed him on a personal level, he said that I was betraying him as a son. He was hurting people . . . he is still hurting people.

The blacks that worked for him in the bottle store, he made them come and tell me that they have no worth, that they were worthless human beings and that I must not trust them. He forced them to do this. He wanted to discourage me from getting involved in politics.

And he is prepared to kill people. He is in with all sorts of commandos. If anything happens to a white family, they are there with their guns. My baby brother is being taught to shoot and take karate lessons. He was forced to take part in the Great Trek thing.

This is so painful to my grandfather whose Jewish parents were killed by the Nazis. My father is half Jewish but now he celebrates Hitler's birthday. My father talks of the 'bloody Jews' who don't love the country and all they want is the money.

I know him, he would not hesitate to kill a black man or what he calls white traitors. He must be tried. I can't go back to that until he is made to face all that he did.

For black members 'return' meant going back to the impoverished black areas that they came from. 'We have no electricity in my home and the water tap is far away.'

The group was also divided between rich and poor. Some members were seen as more fortunate because 'it is not difficult for people with a wealthy family'. The following discussion illustrates this point:

M. (black): He has a brother there, a wealthy brother. Definitely the brother is going to help him.

N. (white): I will tell you what's ready for me when I go back. I have a room, whitewashed, no electricity but I do have a toilet that flushes and some blue-gum trees.

M.: No, I know you have a big house, but that is not the problem. It's more about sharing. Are you prepared to share with people who have nothing? I don't think so.

N.: M., you must remember that I gave all that up because I was not prepared to shed a single drop of blood to protect that big house and all the rest. Don't forget in exile I have been living with very little. I would like to go back, but I am not going to go back on the things that I believe in . . . I would be delighted to share what I have.

Ultimately, the decision to return became a subjective issue. Most of the group members believed that their return was inevitable. This was demonstrated by the continuous mention of 'when I go back'. However, there were the practical constraints such as finding a job, a home and starting all over.

As the possibility of repatriation became more real, growing hostility toward the host country was expressed within the group. Group members felt that they had a country, and were no longer refugees. One member reported that 'In fact I feel a little more equal . . . it's not any more like I am a refugee, a beggar. I belong somewhere . . . I also have a country.' The hostility was often expressed in the group by comparing the Dutch to the Afrikaner. One member said that the Dutch reminded him of some of the 'real' Boers. 'They both have the Calvinistic way of thinking. They don't have any sense of grey, it's yes or no. They have absolutely no sense of nuance in their lives.' Others expressed resentment that 'Dutch society has no easy access, they have a superficial kind of friendliness . . . but in most cases it remains closed.'

Finally, up until the last group meeting none of the group members had made any tentative plans to go back.

## DISCUSSION

The group experience proved to be of great value to the participants, as assessed by statements made during the group discussions
and after termination. 'It broke the isolation. Inevitably one feels
that one represents that collective reputation of the whites. That is
the main thing that I feel has gone. I can trust myself as a person
and not to have to represent white South Africa. I can begin to use
my own mind and trust my own heart in matters. I have a lot of
strength that I did not have before, and I feel that the group has
done that for me. We reached a level of intimacy that was not there
in the community.'

The group not only managed to break down the barriers towards
intimacy and self-disclosure which existed between the members,
but it managed to do this despite the fear of political persecution
among South African refugees. 'Here, in this group,' a black
member said, 'we can go further and look at what we must do to
live together.'

The lessening of feelings of a collective guilt was voiced by a
number of white group members. One expressed his new awareness
eloquently as follows:

The big thing that I learned is the obvious; that I am still 'white'
and you are still 'black' to the eye and that the only borderline
between us is the past. Between you, B., and S., I came clearly
to understand the continuation of the optical prejudice that you
must face and the cold front that you must surpass in order to
live, love and rise up to greet each day. Even though I knew
these things, to hear it said in confidence and trust, destroyed
the barrier of silence that was keeping all of us as
'generalizations'.

The experience of the first moments of being personal, and at
the same time sharing the nature of others, was profound and
delicate at the same time. By profound, I mean real; by delicate,
I mean human, a moment for the heart to know. As the different
obstacles arose and passed, I experienced wonder first, and then

214

shyness. Surely these matters are greater than all of us singly? I cannot help but feel privileged to even be here at all. I was not alone, for this I rejoiced. There were so many present.

The subtle quality that I felt was that of passing from the formal encounter into the heartland of friendship . . . like the passing of a frontier. Certainly these meetings have dispelled the silent curse of not daring to imagine what bad things could be thought of my whiteness in the general reputation that time, truth and treachery bring to light. After being part of those meetings, I am far more at ease in the presence of those 'black people' whom I have not met. I am over the fear of imagining some ugly thing of myself just because I was born a white South African . . .

Another member was more succinct. He said:

I wish to say that my recovery from madness was only possible with the support and help of many people who have suffered the best and the worst of my nature . . . The encounter groups have enabled me to encounter myself, catch myself out and thus instil in me a true sense of confidence and ease with people in general.

The words of a third person, which echo the sentiments of the previous two, conclude this paper. This person said:

I have a lot more strength than I had before, and I feel that this group has done that for me. What has gone is the feeling that I represent the reputation of the whites. I feel that I can trust myself more.

REFERENCES

KUNZ, E. F. (1972), 'The refugee in flight: kinetic models and forms or displacement', *International Migration Review*, 7, 13–25.

MALAN, R. (1990), *My Traitor's Heart*. London: The Bodley Head Press.

MUTISO, R. M. (1979), 'Counselling of refugees in Africa.' Paper presented at Pan African Congress on Refugees, Arusha, Tanzania, in May.

ROGERS, C. (1970), *On Encounter Groups*. London: Harper and Row.

SANFORD, R. (1984), 'The beginning of dialogue in South Africa', *Counseling Psychologist*, 18, 3–14.

SCUDDER, T., and COLSON, E. (1982), 'Conclusion: from welfare to development: a conceptual framework for the analysis of dislocated people', in A. Hansen and A. Oliver-Smith (eds.), *Involuntary Migration and Resettlement*. Boulder: Westview.

STEIN, B. N. (1986), 'The experience of being a refugee: insights from the research literature', in C. L. Williams and J. Westmeyer (eds.), *Refugee Mental Health in Resettlement Countries* (pp. 5–23). Washington: Hemisphere Publishing.

# · 11 ·

# Client-Centred Psychodrama

## JOAO MARQUES-TEIXEIRA

### INTRODUCTION

Psychodrama was invented by Jacob Moreno (Moreno, 1965). He was interested in the crucially important role played by spontaneity in personal growth and, like Rogers, saw group therapy as essentially a process of encounter. Although Rogers and Moreno were very different characters and their approaches to therapy diverged at many points, there is also a tantalizing similarity in their basic concerns. They were also both inspirational figures whose life interest moved from therapy, narrowly conceived, to concern with the good of humankind as a whole.

Recently attempts have been made to develop the common ground between the work of Moreno and Rogers to create a person-centred psychodrama (Hipolito *et al.*, 1986; Brazier, 1991). An extra dimension has sometimes been added by integrating the use of video into the sessions. In this chapter I am making an attempt to explain the implicit structure of such client-centred or person-centred dramatic therapy groups by reference to four 'layers' or 'stages' implicit in the process of such work. The terms 'layer' and 'stage' will be used interchangeably here so that we do not lose track of the fact that while a sequence is generally apparent, each stage or layer, in a sense, also in-dwells in each of the others.

It is important to say at the outset that these four layers are presented here as a means of helping us to make sense of what is going on in such groups. They do not constitute an action plan for how to run them. An actual group may move back and forth between different layers or stages according to its needs. Actually, as we will see, the four stages are an attempt to spell out the implications of a natural movement back and forth between disintegration and reintegration which seems to be an inherent property of any process of change.

Nonetheless, each layer or stratum does tend to have its own language and logic and they tend to form a sequence, each preparing the ground for the next. They thus form both an uninterrupted flow and a kind of functional hierarchy though this is not a hierarchy in the sense of power or authority, nor a sequence which is rigid and invariable. Simply each layer or stage is distinguishable as well as influencing the others. It is also possible to think of the facilitator as functioning as a kind of meta-stratum, attempting to enable clarity, meaning and integration to emerge from the other layers (Fig. 1).

## LAYER ONE: SCENE SETTING

Psychodrama begins with an invitation, explicit or implicit, for members to come forward with scenes they wish to play or offer to the group. Each participant is free to offer something. The group thus has to find a way to organize itself if a single scene is to emerge. There has to be give and take, a dialectic between subjectivity and concern for others, individuation and socialization, as the group seeks a cohesive purpose. This basic structure is therefore an invitation to self-compromise in the interests of the group as a whole.

This first layer of group activity thus has two sub-phases. Firstly, there is the matter of collective self-determination. Members become subjectively aware of the scenes they each can offer which are meaningful to them as individuals and which have the possibility of becoming meaningful to the group as a whole. These are expressed to the group which must then reach a collective consensus about who is to be the protagonist and what scene is to be examined.

The other sub-stage concerns the actual elaboration of a dramatic

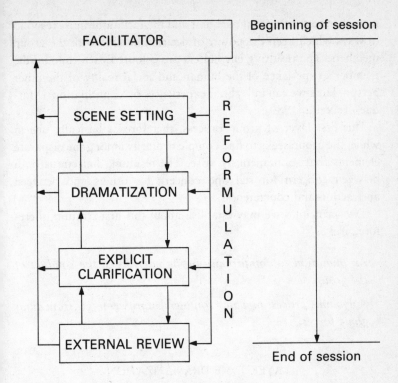

Fig. 1

plot. This includes the creation of characters and definition of a time and place for a scene centred upon the protagonist aided by other group members. In this activity thought and imagination are both required in a co-ordinated way. What has been subjective to one group member must now be concretely represented to and by all the group members. As the scene unfolds, there is also a qualitative jump from verbal communication to dramatic dialogue.

Generally the protagonist takes a central part at this stage, choosing and distributing roles among the participants including him or herself. There is thus a process of giving and receiving by group members which makes greater demands upon each member than is common in many groups. If the group is to remain person-centred, the group members must all have freedom to involve themselves in this process even though the protagonist will, necessarily,

219

have the most influential part in it and the facilitator must respond in ways which keep the power of decision making with the group members. The resulting encounters are coloured each time by the member's experience of the human and social reality of the other person. Here we can talk about experiences of 'confirmation' (Marques-Teixeira, 1989).

This first layer of group process, therefore, is basically one in which the group seeks to find complementarity among the disparate elements that spontaneously arise. The resulting dialectic is both between concern for self and concern for others and between abstraction and concreteness.

Two principles we may establish about this first stratum, therefore, are:

*An invitation to compromise in the interests of the conduct of the group.*

*A dynamic process in which complementarity emerges from antagonic forces.*

## LAYER TWO: DRAMATIZATION

This is the heart of the method. Dramatization through the playing of scenes is the hallmark of the psychodrama method. The main characteristic of the work is that it consists of dramatic action evolving in its own time and space and according to its own inherent logic. It is as though a special inner space is created within the field of the group. In this special space there can be play and fantasy.

This kind of drama allows maximal approach of the individual to their imaginary personal world of wish and fantasy. It also allows individuals to escape from their habitual mode of being. A person who expresses himself in the role of another: 'I am not myself, but another speaks through me,' expands his imagination and himself. This expansion could be regarded as an internal dialectic, a self-generating process of growth. There is a paradox here, too. Authenticity grows out of the experience of being something other than oneself.

Drama does not obey the principles of logic and rationalism. It follows the rhythm of poetry. The constant subtle shifts in dramatic action allow metamorphosis. Codes and stereotypes provide a beginning, but they then lose their rigidity as the group members play with them. Actors can experiment with distancing from and identifying with real and imaginary parts.

Two principles relating to this stage, therefore, are:

*Growth through simultaneously being oneself and being another.*

*Discovering the emergent properties of free dramatic enactment.*


## LAYER THREE: EXPLICIT CLARIFICATION

Having surrendered themselves to the flow of spontaneous creativity in the dramatization with all its imagery and prompts to expanded awareness, there now comes the necessity of trying to clarify what has happened. Each actor and participant now has the opportunity to express feelings or elaborate upon what has taken place. The imagination is still working as the group seeks to find ways of understanding and integrating what has taken place.

Also, at this stage, the group has to knit together not only what took place in the second phase, that is, in the dramatization; it also has to integrate phases one and two. In the wake of dramatization, therefore, there is a need to pull together the work of imagination which people have shared and the real relations which they have with each other. This leads to a more and more complex group interaction. Yet out of this can come an enhanced clarity for each individual as they regard themselves as persons in role, in life and in relation to the group.

So this phase is also one of reorganization. What has happened over these first three phases is that creative possibilities have been shared, then worked with and elaborated and now reintegrated.

This is a movement through temporary disorganization toward the emergence of new clarity.

Principles relevant to this phase are:

*There is a natural actualizing tendency at work in the process of the group.*

*Out of complexity emerges new order.*


## LAYER FOUR: REVIEWING FROM OUTSIDE

The effectiveness of psychodrama, like any phenomenological method, rests upon the fact that we can gain new insight by changing our perspective. In psychodrama this is often achieved by role reversal with other players. The use of video permits a further twist to this process by allowing the whole group to stand outside their work and re-view it. This is a figure-ground inversion, a gestalt movement, which enables the participants to see themselves now from the outside.

The process of viewing a video of a piece of dramatic enactment which, in the first place, arose spontaneously, also involves stages of disintegration and reintegration as the group take apart what they have done and then put it back together again in their minds. The act of trying to understand involves dividing the work up into analysable parts, only to find that no part can be understood in isolation from the whole.

Moreno invented psychodrama as a method in which the audience could take over the stage and instead of watching heroes and villains being portrayed to them, could become their own characters. The use of video allows the further role reversal in which they can return to their seats to view themselves, but now do so from a position of power.

## PERSON-CENTRED PRINCIPLES IN PSYCHODRAMA

I have evolved a model, based upon research done with a client-centred psychodrama group run over 37 weeks, of the way in which person-centred principles become effective in groups using dramatic methods. This research involved the use of questionnaires to measure the anxiety levels, depression and self-concepts of clients before, during and after therapy, and also other questionnaires to achieve some measurement of facilitators' attitudes and characteristics of the process of the group itself.

This research suggested that the clients in question had indeed made progress in reducing their symptoms of depression and anxiety and that they had also changed their views of themselves in more global ways. Research on a single group can never be conclusive but these results were encouraging. The good results for participants were thus both specific and global.

In line with what is predicted by person-centred principles (Rogers, 1957), this work suggested that the exhibition of qualities of empathy, congruence and unconditional regard by the facilitator promoted group cohesiveness directly and that it also fostered co-operative relationships between members and made the process of getting into dramatization easier.

These relationships can be summarized in a diagram (Fig.2).

## CONCLUSIONS

There is some common ground between Moreno and Rogers and in this space there is room to create a genuinely person-centred action-based therapy. This method may, in due course, evolve in its own way and grow beyond its roots.

The person-centred approach tends to favour unstructured work while psychodrama works from a structure toward spontaneity. We have tried to show here that the structures used by psychodramatists, however, are better regarded as part of a natural progression which does not have to be organized by the worker but evolves

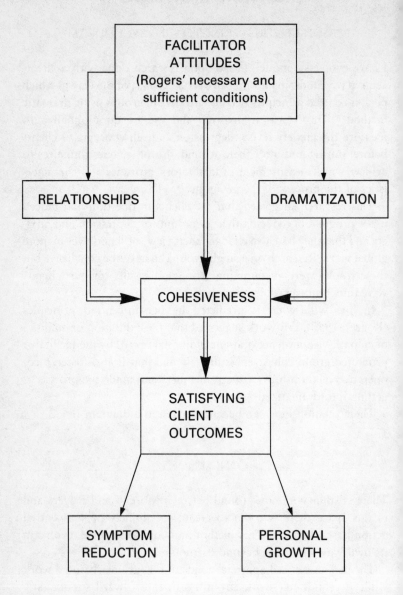

Fig. 2

anew whenever a group makes a serious attempt to use action-based methods.

At a cognitive level, growth is a matter of alternating phases of disintegration and reintegration. At an action level, growth is a matter of metamorphosis through surrendering oneself to the spontaneously emergent qualities, or what might more easily be called the poetry, of the situation. To pull these two principles together I have offered a four-layer model of what is going on in a person-centred psychodrama group.

Finally, I have suggested that good outcomes for participants are enhanced by the cohesiveness which comes from a group having been involved in action together as well as simply talk. The core conditions of empathy, congruence and unconditional positive regard offered by the group facilitator not only contribute directly to this cohesiveness, they also help to create the atmosphere of safety in which a group can undertake the kinds of dramatization which seem to amplify the power of their interactions with one another.

This amplifying effect found in dramatization seems to be to do with the fact that drama, especially when videoed and reviewed, enables a group to achieve a higher order of complexity in their interrelations with one another, out of which a higher order or reintegration becomes possible.

REFERENCES

BRAZIER, D. J. (1991), *A Guide to Psychodrama*. London: Association for Humanistic Psychology.

HIPOLITO, J., COELHO, F., GARCIA, R., GODINHO, J., and NUNES, O. (1986), 'Experiencia de dois Grupos de Psicodrama: perspectiva antropoanalitica.' Paper presented at the 2nd Congresso Nacional de Psiquiatria Social, Lisboa, Portugal.

MARQUES-TEIXEIRA, J. (1989), 'O Psicodrama na perspectiva da Abordagem Centrada na Pessoa', *O Medico*, 121, 75–94.

MORENO, J. L. (1965), *Psychotherapie de Groupe et Psychodrame.* Paris: PUF.

ROGERS, C. (1957), 'The necessary and sufficient conditions of therapeutic personality change', *Journal of Consulting Psychology,* 21, 95–103.

# Part 3

## *Towards the Future*

· 12 ·

# Can We Afford not to Revision the Person-centred Concept of Self?

## LEN HOLDSTOCK

### INTRODUCTION

During the past decade the focus on the individual as the unit of the social order has come in for widespread criticism. This shift in emphasis accompanies the transition from the modern to the postmodern era and the development toward a globally linked world system (Sampson, 1989a). According to Geertz (1974) the 'Western concept of the person as a bounded, unique, more or less integrated motivational and cognitive universe, a dynamic center of awareness, emotion, judgement and action organized into a distinctive whole and set contrastively both against other such wholes and against its social and natural background, is, however incorrigible it may seem to us, a rather peculiar idea within the context of the world's cultures' (p. 275).

Apart from being described as monocultural, the approach to the self as a demarcated entity has also been depicted as ethnocentric (Hermans, Kempen and van Loon, in press); rationalistic, individualistic, and monotheistic (Johnson, 1985); egocentric (Sampson, 1985; Shweder and Bourne, 1989); a centralized equilibrium structure (Sampson, 1985); self-contained (Sampson, 1988); bounded (Geertz, 1974); individuocentric (Jahoda, 1988); self-reliant and independent (Spence, 1985). Somewhat more critical have been descriptions of the self as bourgeois (Sampson, 1989b; Slugoski and Ginsburg, 1989), selfish (Schwartz, 1986), and empty (Cushman, 1990).

It is in the context of such views that the self-concept underlying

229

the person-centred approach of Carl Rogers (1959, 1977), needs to be evaluated. Since its inception the self-actualizing and self-directing qualities of people have been basic assumptions of the person-centred approach. The point of departure of the person-centred approach has remained firmly embedded in the centrality of the self and the autonomy of the individual. 'The origin of control resided inside the person rather than within the larger system or field' (Holdstock, 1990a, p. 110). Even in the social outreach of the theory, empowering the individual remained the focus through which societal change was thought to be brought about.

This chapter reviews the contemporary emergence within divergent disciplines of alternative models of self which may, in time, serve as a basis for a thoroughly revisioned person-centred concept. It hints at the possibility of a concept of the person which challenges the monocultural notion of the self as a demarcated entity, set off against the world. In this newer view, the self is considered to be inextricably intertwined with other people. The extended concept of the self may even include the deceased as well as the larger universe of animals, plants and inanimate objects. Power and control are not considered to rest predominantly with the individual but within the field of forces within which the individual exists (Holdstock, 1990b).

## A BRIEF HISTORICAL JOURNEY

For many centuries philosophers, novelists and poets have reflected on the nature of the self. Among the philosophers Descartes, Locke, Hume, Kant, and Sartre are of the most prominent ones who 'have addressed themselves to the issue of what must logically be postulated to explain the unity, continuity, and self-sameness in man' (Slugoski and Ginsberg, 1989, p. 36).

Among the literary immortals feature Shakespeare, Hesse, Blake, e.e. cummings, Thoreau and others. However, it was with publication of *The Principles of Psychology* in 1890 that William James first explicated the self-concept in psychology. His distinction between 'the self as knower' (I) and 'the self as known' (the empirical Self, or Me), continues to form the basis of current work in the area. It also provides an appropriate framework with which to approach the person-centred concept of self.

Of the various philosophers, the work of Hegel in particular seems to have played a major role in shaping the ideas of James (van der Veer, 1985). According to Hegel, 'the individual self was in no sense immediately given, but a socially created concept. One cannot have self-consciousness without the 'mediation' of other people . . . It is thus in Hegel's opinion absurd to believe that there is an individual self prior to the interaction with other people . . . The emphasis on the interaction with other people is in Hegel's philosophy connected with the view of active individuals . . . For Hegel to know was also to be engaged in an activity' (van der Veer, 1985, p. 7).

The influence of Hegel is not only to be found in the work of James, but through James, and also directly, in many writings on the self-concept during the past century. Among these theories are those of the symbolic interactionists (Mead, 1968), the social constructionists (see Gordon and Gergen, 1968), cognitive (Kelly, 1955; Rotter, 1954) and other personality theorists (Allport, 1937), as well as sociologists (Marx, Engels, Parsons, Durkheim, Weber, and Sorokin). The idea of a self which is constructed in interaction with others has recently been amplified to include the historical and socio-economic-political context within which interaction occurs (Gergen, 1989; Harré, 1989; Sampson, 1989b).

Of special interest are developments within such diverse disciplines as philosophy and the human movement sciences, which stress the importance of the self as agent in relation (Dokecki, 1990; Holdstock, 1991). The human movement sciences provide an appropriate umbrella for elaborating the activity component without which the self cannot be known. The self emerges in what we do or do not do, and in how we behave towards each other.

## CONSTRUCTIONIST PERSPECTIVES

The thinking of James (1890/1950) that a person 'has as many different social selves as there are distinct *groups* of persons about whose opinion he cares' (p. 179), was continued in the work of the symbolic interactionists (Mead, 1968) and later the social constructionists (see Gordon and Gergen, 1968).

The symbolic interactionists maintained that the self, and all other higher psychological processes, developed through social interaction. The social act was the unit around which the self-concept was formed. It was through communicative interaction that the individual gained information about the attitude of others towards him or herself. 'And it is this generalized other in his experience which provides him with a self' (Mead, 1968, p. 58). 'Once an individual's self has become objectified in the contexts of particular courses of social conduct, this self serves as one basis of control over that individual's future conduct' (Gordon and Gergen, 1968, p. 34).

It is clear from the thinking of the symbolic interactionists that the self was constituted in a larger totality. While the self-as-experienced, the *Me* in James' terminology, became multifaceted, the self-as-experiencer, the *I*, remained nuclear, though. Elaboration of the multifaceted nature of the 'I' had to await developments in cognitive psychology.

## COGNITIVE PERSPECTIVES

Through 'the selective industry of the mind', James (1890/1950, p. 310) believed that our self-feeling was in our power. The 'doing' side of personality, the Self as Knower, the I, 'that which at any moment is conscious' (James, 1892, p. 195), was emphasized by Rotter (1954) and Kelly (1955). The work of these two psychologists facilitated the transformation towards the cognitive perspective which is of such prominence in the psychology of the self at present (Epstein, 1973; Cantor, 1990).

Rotter (1954) pointed out that people made choices by construing situations, tasks, or problems in a certain way. Kelly (1955) carried the analysis a step further. According to him each individual was a naïve scientist, actively functioning in terms of personal constructs about the self and the social world. Indeed, the cognitive self has become firmly established as the captain of our souls and the master of our fate.

More recently, various models have been proposed to conceptualize the self in terms of self-schemas, scripts, and prototypes (Markus and Wurff, 1987). It would appear that the pendulum has begun to swing towards the 'self as a process rather than a thing' (Gordon, 1968, p. 136), as William James would have liked us to consider the I. However, attention remains focused 'on the individual's active attempts to understand the world, to take control, and to reach personal goals. At the heart of this approach is a strong respect for the power of cognition to generate choice or to create freedom. Individuals overcome stimulus control at least in part by giving their own meaning to events, by cognitively transforming situations' (Cantor, 1990, p. 736).

Markus and Wurff (1987), similarly, propose a 'working self-concept' with both stable and malleable characteristics. Rogers (1959) did not formulate his concept of self in cognitive terms. In fact he tended to view experiencing, which is such a core component of the self-concept, as a rather passive process. However, Wexler (1974) indicated quite clearly that experiencing is created by actively processing available information.

In summary, the main contribution of the constructionist and cognitive perspectives has been that it highlighted the multifaceted nature of the self-as-experienced (*Me*) and the self-as-experiencer (*I*). Both the *Me* and the *I* became multifaceted. However, the multiple selves, whether of Me or I, continued to be considered within a centralized self-concept. In the terminology of William James (1892), one nuclear self continued to encompass not only many social selves but also a continuously changing stream of consciousness.

However, in the most recent thinking along constructionist lines the self is basically considered to be dialogical. The 'dialogical self has the character of a decentralized, polyphonic narrative with a multiplicity of *I*-positions' (Hermans, Kempen, and van Loon, in press, p. 22). Hermans and his co-workers consider the self to be a dialogical narrator, '(a) spatially organized and *embodied* and (b) social, with the other not outside but *in* the self-structure, resulting in a multiplicity of dialogically interacting selves. The embodied nature of the self contrasts with conceptions of a disembodied or "rationalistic" mind' (p. 3).

In essence, an embodied self-concept, with the other not outside but incorporated in the self-structure, seems to me what the person-centred approach is essentially about. And yet, in the theory under-lying the approach, the self continues to be regarded as an autonomous entity. It is considered sufficient for the world of the other to be entered in an as-if way. The therapist only takes up a position in the client's frame of reference. The other is not con-sidered to be an essential part of the therapist, or the therapist part of the other. Whether persons who function within the person-centred framework are capable of transcending or limiting their theatrical distance, is an open question. The embeddedness of the person-centred approach in the cultural context of a bounded, highly centralized self will undoubtedly make incorporation of the other in the self very difficult. Apart from the developments outlined above, the following sources of critique of the nuclear self need to be considered.

## REFLECTIONS FROM WITHIN THE FEMALE PERSPECTIVE

'Feminist reconceptualizations of the patriarchical version of social, historical and psychological life have introduced some strikingly different views of personhood' (Sampson, 1989b, p. 2). Several feminist and post-feminist writers have proposed an alternative to the autonomous and non-relational model of the self. According to them the emphasis on the separation-individuation side of identity reflects the male perspective. The female perspective refers to ' "the other voice" with which many women seem to confront the world and in terms of which they frame their understanding. This is the voice of connections and relationships rather than the voice of boundaries and separations' (Sampson, 1988, p. 18). 'Women move along in the world through relational connections . . . The notion of a separate identity or a separate sense of self is not quite the same in women as in men' (Josselson, 1987, pp. 169–70).

According to Josselson (1987) women never set themselves as sharply apart from others because of their early developmental history. The factor which is of crucial importance in early development is the unique nature of the mother–daughter relationship. Because the mother as primary love object is the same gender as the daughter, identification does not require such drastic separation as in the case of boys. In order to identify himself as a male with father, the boy must pull himself away from his primary attachment to the mother. 'As a result, girls experience themselves as being more continuous with others . . . Boundaries of the self are never as rigid in girls as in boys, and the basic female sense of self is connected, with a good deal of fluidity, to the world' (Josselson, 1987, p. 170). Josselson also states that due to gender similarities the mother's investment in the daughter is likely to be more intense and to last longer than her investment in her son.

Thus women grow up with a relational sense of self. Identity means 'being with'. Without others there is no sense of a fulfilled self. The more there is of others the more there is of self, and vice versa. Identity seems to be a matter of defining the internal experience of the self through attachment to others. Unlike males who are brought up in a culture stressing self-assertion, mastery, individual distinction, and separateness, what Bakan (1966) called *agency*, women are raised in a culture of *communion*, stressing contact, union, co-operation, and being together. For many women communion is more important than agency. To be related, is itself an expression of agentic needs for assertion, mastery, and achievement. Skill and success in relatedness becomes keystones of identity.

Josselson (1990) discusses seven dimensions of relationship as foundations and expressions of identity. According to her the needs for holding, attachment, and libidinal gratification are the most basic. The first two needs are self-explanatory. In the third, the libido is object and not pleasure-seeking. Falling in love is opening up to another person(s). Passion is such an intensely affirming experience because of the unity which is achieved in the physical bonding. The fourth dimension is that of being affirmed or negated by others. One needs to be affirmed. However hard we try to live independently of another's affirmation, being mirrored in another's validation affords one the opportunity to find oneself. Experiences of being affirmed or negated by others are an integral part of the intersubjective context of identity.

The same is true of the fifth dimension of relatedness, idealization and identification. According to Josselson (1990) adolescents need to have heroes. She considers adolescents who cannot admire to be at risk. As her sixth dimension of identity she regards embeddedness as being of vital importance. Identity emerges from the groups in which one is embedded. It is the soil in which identity grows. The self is part of the social world and the social world is part of the self. The *We* of *Me* conveys the intimate linkage of the self to the social world.

Finally, identity emerges from what one offers to others in the form of care. Tenderness and care are seldom talked about in terms of identity. It simply is not part of the developmental ethic which we hold as important in raising our children. This is especially true in the socialization of boys. Elsewhere I have written that 'Boys should be exposed to the same training that girls traditionally receive in our society, and should be encouraged to develop similar kinds of socially positive, tender, co-operative, nurturing, and sensitive qualities' (Holdstock, 1990c). Perhaps relatedness is not only central to identity in women; perhaps it is also of central importance to the identity of males, even though males do not quite realize just how much, geared as they are to the language of power and assertion (Josselson, 1990). 'Our developmental psychology, as well as our culture, has tended to equate maturity with independence and impenetrable personal boundaries, thus relegating the interpenetration of selves in relatedness to a less mature form of existence' (Josselson, 1987, p. 185). We should strive to make heroic the achievement of intimacy and care. Skills in this regard certainly do not detract from functioning effectively in any work situation.

## THE CHALLENGE TO LIBERAL INDIVIDUALISM

Liberal individualism gives people the right to their own lives so long as this does not intrude on the lives of others. People are not considered to derive identities and human capacities from their membership in any particular social order. They, as individuals, take precedence (MacIntyre, 1988). By viewing individuals as prior to society, the liberal ethic 'fails to offer a blueprint for the era of globalization in which persons will increasingly be part of a thoroughly linked, interdependent global world system. Actions in one segment of this system have consequences for all, and therefore a more constitutive vision is required' (Sampson, 1989a, p. 919).

> ... the human race to be shown as one great network or tissue which quivers in every part when one point is shaken, like a spider's web if touched.
>
> Thomas Hardy, *The Dynasts*

## CRITICAL THEORY

Critical theory raises the ideological implications of psychology's focus on the individual as a relatively autonomous and distinctive unit. Sampson (1985) pointed out that the 'democratic political ideal we hope to achieve is contradicted by the personhood ideal we espouse' (p. 1207). The self as a 'distinctive universe is said to reflect the sham and the illusion that is the bourgeois individual, not its reality' (Sampson, 1989b, p. 3). Socio-economic and political forces not only dictate what is possible, but also shape the ideology concerning individuality which is necessary to maintain and perpetuate the status quo. The focus on individual psychotherapy rather than on societal ills is a case in point (Albee, 1982, 1986; Prilleltensky, 1989; Sarason, 1981).

Due to his contribution to the field of psychotherapy, Rogers has been the target of a great deal of criticism (see Holdstock, 1990a for references). For instance, Sarason (1981) argued that by defining the problems of people in personal and narrowly interpersonal terms, independent of the nature and structure of the social order, Rogers created a stumbling block to the solution of mental health problems. Despite being looked on as a quiet revolutionary, Rogers was firmly locked into the ideology of his own indigenous culture.

## DEVELOPMENTS IN VARIOUS SCIENTIFIC DISCIPLINES

Developments in various scientific disciplines indicate an holistic order underlying the physical universe (e.g. Bentov, 1977; Wilber, 1984; Young, 1986). The rediscovery of Smuts' (1926) *Holism and Evolution* has drawn attention to the invisible but powerful organizing principle, nature's drive to synthesize, which is operative in the universe. It is proposed that if we did not look at wholes we would fail to understand the structure and functioning of the universe. Holism also finds expression in the General Systems Theory of Ludwig von Bertalanffy (1969). General Systems Theory, more recently expounded by Laszlo (1972), sees all of nature, including human behaviour, as interconnected. Nothing can be understood in isolation, but must be seen as part of a system. The influence of holism and General Systems Theory is evident in many disciplines, including psychology. Unfortunately the psychological derivative does not acknowledge its historical connectedness to holism and to General Systems Theory. Even Lewin's (1951) Field Theory already seems to have been forgotten. Field Theory granted primacy to relationships rather than to individual entities, and pointed to a self which was constituted in a larger totality, as did symbolic interactionism.

Both the unitive dimension, which is such a key concept of General Systems Theory, and holism have recently been elaborated further by Nobel Laureate David Bohm (in Wilber, 1982) and by the neuropsychologist Karl Pribram (in press). In his Unified Field Theory Bohm suggests that the organization of the universe may be holographic. He further suggests that what we normally regard as reality is only the explicit, or unfolded order of things. Bohm recognizes an implicate, or enfolded order which underlies this apparent reality. The implicate order harbours reality in much the same way that the DNA is the nucleus of the cell harbours potential life and directs the nature of its unfolding. According to the holonomic view of Pribram the 'I' is enfolded in the whole and every part of the whole contributes to the individual 'I'. At the same time the individual 'I' contributes to and contains something of the whole. Thus each individual and each culture is contained in an implicitly enfolded order. Within the spiral of time and perturbations of the socio-economic-political-cultural-physical environment the enfolded universe unfolds. Individual and cultural differences manifest as aspects of the unfolded reality.

> Man's body and proud brain are mosaics of the same elemental particles that compose the dark, drifting clouds of interstellar space.
>
> Lincoln Barnett

Another scientific development with profound implications for theories about the self is Prigogine's work in nonequilibrium physics, for which he received the Nobel prize in 1977. A detailed discussion of this work is not possible here, but interested readers are referred to Ferguson (1980) for an introduction and to *Order Out of Chaos* (Prigogine and Stengers, 1984) for an advanced discussion. In essence, nonequilibrium theory suggests that the self does not derive its order from being a closed, singular and thoroughly integrated system, but rather from being an open system which is involved in a continuous exchange of energy with the environment.

239

## MAINSTREAM PSYCHOLOGY

A lively debate has ensued in the *American Psychologist*, the official organ of the American Psychological Association, concerning the monocultural orientation and exclusive focus on the autonomous individual in psychology (e.g. Albee, 1982, 1986; Bandura, 1982; Corlett, 1988; Cushman, 1990; Dansereau, 1989; Gibbs and Schnell, 1985; Ho, 1985; Hogan, 1975; Perloff, 1987; Prilleltensky, 1989; Sampson, 1985, 1989a; Sarason, 1981; Spence, 1985; Waterman, 1981). This debate reflects the growing awareness within mainstream psychology that alternative realities to the ones with which it is familiar, do exist.

## TRANSCULTURAL PERSPECTIVES

A campaign against the ethnocentric, Western view of self has also been launched in many other disciplines in the social sciences. Alternative concepts of self which are inextricably embedded in the framework of society, culture and time have been presented. The issue is not simply one of the multiple social roles of the self which James and many others since have acknowledged, but a totally different notion of what constitutes the self.

Cultural and psychological anthropology (Hallowell, 1976), transcultural psychiatry (Kleinman, 1980), cross-cultural (Bond, 1988) and indigenous psychologies (Diaz-Guerrero, 1977; Heelas and Lock, 1981) provide a wealth of information which argues against the monocultural individuocentric approach to the self. Anthropologists have made a clear distinction between universalist and cultural relativist expositions of the self in order to clarify the apparent diversity of human understandings. Universalists claim that the basic psychological processes are the same for people all over the world. They allege, for example, that the concept of reward has the same reinforcing properties for all people, and that schizophrenia manifests in all cultures. 'Apparently different but really the same', is the universalist slogan. Equality and homogeneity take precedence over diversity. An intriguing universalist concept, as expressed by Malpass (1988), is that 'individuals in Western nations adequately represent human populations everywhere. This is because we share certain life processes and environmental demands with human populations everywhere' (p. 29). According to Malpass it is debatable whether there is 'any evidence of real differences in cognitive or other psychological processes across cultures' (p. 31).

Cultural relativists believe that there is ample evidence of such differences. They argue that the effect of culture is too great to maintain universality of principles and their slogan is 'Different but equal'. The extreme exponents of cultural relativism argue that what is valid in one culture is invalid everywhere else. However, Triandis (1988) suggests that it is more appropriate to consider psychological attributes to be of relative universal validity. The principle of reinforcement would thus have high universal validity, whereas the principle of self as a self-contained unit would have low universal validity. Therefore, 'Whereas all cultures recognize the individual as empirical agent, most agents do not retain the individualistic conceptions of the person' (Miller, 1988, p. 275). Indigenous psychologies 'often have very different and more socially orientated notions of what constitutes a person' (Jahoda, 1988, p. 91). The other and society are not only of importance in establishing a concept of self, as the symbolic interactionists and social constructionists emphasized, or in providing the context within which social roles are to be enacted, but are also integral components of the self.

## THE SELF IN NON-WESTERN CULTURES

The basic unit in non-Western culture is a 'bi-polar self-other relationship . . . born out of the social or sharing process' (Kohlberg in Gibbs and Schnell, 1985, p. 1074). Shweder and Bourne (1989) described the bipolar self as sociocentric-organic in contrast to the egocentric-contractual self of the West. 'Linked to each other in an interdependent system, members of organic cultures take an active interest in one another's affairs, and feel at ease regulating and being regulated' (Shweder and Bourne, 1989, p. 132). 'The self tends to be conceived as inherently social and as permeable, if not constituted, by contextual influences' (Miller, 1988, p. 273).

The self in non-Western cultures has been defined both in terms of the nature of the self-nonself boundary and also in terms of the location of power and control (Heelas and Lock, 1981). Thus, terms such as field control and a decentralized non-equilibrium structure (Sampson, 1985) have been used to distinguish the non-Western attitude towards the self.

There are 'wide variations in what counts as the self' (Tedeschi, 1988, p. 19) among non-Western cultures. To make sense of this variety, individualism-collectivism has been singled out as the major dimension of cultural variability by many theorists, collectivist cultures being those where 'group memberships are more important for self-conceptions ... than in individualistic cultures' (Gudykunst, 1988, p. 169).

The following cultures, listed in alphabetical order, 'each portray the self as constituted by social context rather than by an individuated psychological core' (Miller, 1988, p. 273): African (Akbar, 1984; Asante, 1983; Baldwin, 1986; Holdstock, 1987); Balinese (Geertz, 1974); Cheyene (Miller, 1988); Chewong of Malaysia (Howell, 1981); Chinese (Ho, 1985; Hsu, 1985; Tuan, 1982; Weiming, 1985; Yang, 1988); Gahuku-Gama of New Guinea (see Shweder and Bourne, 1989); Indian (Bharati, 1985; Miller, 1988; Shweder and Bourne, 1989; Sinha, 1984); Inuit (Eskimo) (Harré, 1981); Islamic (Harré, 1981); Japanese (Azuma, 1984a, b; De Vos, 1985; Doi in Johnson, 1985; Kimura, 1971; Kojima, 1984); Javanese (Geertz, 1974); Lohorung of eastern Nepal (Hardman, 1981); Maori (Harré, 1981; Smith, 1981); Moroccan (Geertz, 1974); Ojibwa Indians of Northern America (Hallowell, 1976); and the Zapotec of Mexico (see Shweder and Bourne, 1989).

Even if the universalist position has to be abandoned, a common factor would appear to underlie the approach to self in most of the world's cultures. This common factor seems to be the sociocentric or embedded self, and not the bounded, masterful self. Nevertheless, the West, in its study of the self, has set its own standards as universal criteria, just as it has in many other areas. Furthermore, a wide range of opinions exists within those cultures which hold a sociocentric conceptualization of the self. It is evident that the cultures mentioned inhabit widespread geographical environments, and that there can be cultural variations within even one geographical region. In addition, when considering the way the self is conceptualized, account must be taken of such variables as modernization (Triandis, 1988), hierarchical group membership (e.g. caste and social class) (Gudykunst, 1988) and the dominance of the masculine aspect within a culture (Hofstede, 1980).

In many cultures, such as the African and Maori cultures, the fluidity of the self-other boundary does not pertain only to the individual, to the family and to society, but also to the physical universe and metaphysical reality. In other societies, for example those of India, this fluidity acknowledges the world of other people, but focuses primarily on the relationship with the metaphysical. Whereas Hinduism accentuates the immutable self to the extent that the individual self is regarded as an illusion, Chinese Confucianism establishes the person, and hence the self, centrally within the community of others. Inuit culture shows a similarity to Hinduism in that the importance of the individual is curtailed. At the same time, it shows a similarity to Confucianism in its emphasis on the importance of the individual's role as part of a community (DeVos, Marsella and Hsu, 1985; Shweder and Bourne, 1989).

The self seems to have travelled a long way since the time of William James. However, if we are to build on James' farsighted vision we need to take non-Western conceptualizations of the self into account, even though they are not recognized in the formalized contexts with which the West is familiar. Poincare (in Jahoda, 1988) refers to the importance of astronomy and geology in furthering our understanding of the physical world. He states:

> By making long excursions in space and time, we find our ordinary rules completely upset, and these great upsettings will give us a clearer view and a better comprehension of such small

changes as may occur nearer us, in the small corner of the world in which we are called to live and move. We shall know this corner better for the journey we have taken into distant lands where we had no concern (p. 95).


## SUMMARY

As we approach the end of this century and prepare to enter a new era, it is necessary to take stock of some of the implicit assumptions which underlie the discipline and the profession of psychology. One of these implicit assumptions is the belief that it is as a self-contained and autonomous entity that the individual serves as the central unit of society.

Since its inception, person-centred theory has subscribed to this core assumption. In fact the uniqueness of the person-centred approach has been its emphasis on the subjective nature of the individual's experience, on the self-actualizing and self-directing qualities of people. The notion of empowering the person, trusting the person to know the proper direction of movement in her or his own actualizing process, is one of the fundamental aspects of the theory. Even in the social outreach of the theory, each individual remained the focus through which societal change was thought to be achieved.

However, postmodern developments towards a globally linked world system call for a dramatic revisioning of the way the self has been conceptualized. Within these developments the prevailing concept or self has been described as monocultural, monotheistic, analytic, rationalistic, individualistic, individuocentric and egocentric, as well as a centralized equilibrium structure, bourgeois, and empty.

Reaction to the individuocentric model of the self has emanated from divergent sources. Among these have been: feminist and post-feminist writings; critical theory; deconstructionism; social interactionism; developments in the natural sciences which can be summarized under the notions of holism, field theory, general systems theory, and unified field theory; developments in sociology, social, cross-cultural and even mainstream psychology; cultural and psychological anthropology; transcultural psychiatry; and the developing indigenous psychologies.

The alternative model of the self, which emanates from the sources above, challenges the notion of the self as a demarcated entity, set off against the world. Power and control are not considered to rest predominantly with the individual, but within the field of forces within which the individual exists. This 'new' concept of self has also been described as sociocentric-organic, bipolar, communal, open, ensembled, a decentralized nonequilibrium structure, polytheistic, pluralistic, holistic, and dialogical.

The major task confronting humanity is to create a new self, better suited than the model adhered to at present by psychology, in order to deal with the issues of our global and postmodern society. Whether person-centred theory can rise to the challenge of revisioning its individuocentric approach to the self remains an open question.

REFERENCES

AKBAR, N. (1984), 'Africentric social sciences for human liberation', *Journal of Black Studies*, 14, 395–414.

ALBEE, G. W. (1982), 'Preventing psychopathology and promoting human potential', *American Psychologist*, 37, 1043–50.

ALBEE, G. W. (1986), 'Toward a just society: lessons from observations on the primary prevention of psychopathology', *American Psychologist*, 41, 891–98.

ALLPORT, G. W. (1937), *Personality: a psychological interpretation*. New York: Holt.

ASANTE, M. K. (1983), 'The ideological significance of Afrocentricity in inter-cultural communication', *Journal of Black Studies*, 14, 3–19.

AZUMA, H. (1984a), 'Secondary control as a heterogeneous category', *American Psychologist*, 39, 970–71.

AZUMA, H. (1984b), 'Psychology in a non-Western country', *International Journal of Psychology*, 19, 45–55.

BAKAN, D. (1966), *The Duality of Human Existence*. Chicago: Rand McNally.

BALDWIN, J. A. (1986), 'African (Black) psychology: issues and synthesis', *Journal of Black Studies*, 16, 235–49.

BANDURA, A. (1982), 'Self-efficacy mechanism in human agency', *American Psychologist*, 37, 122–47.

BENTOV, I. (1977), *Stalking the Wild Pendulum*. New York: Dutton.

BHARATI, A. (1985), 'The self in Hindu thought and action', in A. J. Marsella, G. DeVos, and F. L. K. Hsu (eds.), *Culture and Self: Asian and Western perspectives* (pp. 185–230). London: Tavistock.

BOND, M. H. (ed.), (1988), *The Cross-Cultural Challenge to Social Psychology*. London: Sage.

CANTOR, N. (1990), 'From thought to behavior: "Having" and "doing" in the study of personality and cognition', *American Psychologist*, 45, 735–50.

CORLETT, J. A. (1988), 'Perloff, utilitarianism, and existentialism: problems with self-interest and personal responsibility', *American Psychologist*, 43, 481–83.

CUSHMAN, P. (1990), 'Why the self is empty: toward a historically situated psychology', *American Psychologist*, 45, 599–611.

DANSEREAU, F. (1989), 'A multiple level of analysis perspective on the debate about individualism', *American Psychologist*, 44, 959–60.

DEVOS, G. (1985), 'Dimensions of the self in Japanese culture', in A. J. Marsella, G. DeVos, and F. L. K. Hsu (eds.), *Culture and Self: Asian and Western perspectives* (pp. 141–84). London: Tavistock.

DEVOS, G., MARSELLA, A. J., and HSU, F. L. K. (1985), 'Introduction: approaches to culture and self', in G. DeVos, A. J. Marsella, and F. L. K. Hsu (eds.), *Culture and Self: Asian and Western perspectives* (pp. 2–23). London: Tavistock.

DIAZ-GUERRERO, R. (1977), 'A Mexican psychology', *American Psychologist*, 32, 934–44.

DOKECKI, P. R. (1990), 'On knowing the person as agent in caring relations', *Person-Centered Review*, 5, 155–69.

EPSTEIN, S. (1973), 'The self-concept revisited: or a theory of a theory', *American Psychologist*, 28, 404–16.

FERGUSON, M. (1980), *The Aquarian Conspiracy*. Los Angeles: J. P. Tarcher.

GEERTZ, C. (1974), '"From the nature's point of view": on the nature of anthropological understanding', in K. Basso and H. Selby (eds.), *Meaning in Anthropology* (pp. 221–37). Albuquerque: University of New Mexico Press.

GERGEN, K. J. (1989), 'Warranting voice and the elaboration', in J. Shotter and K. J. Gergen (eds.), *Texts of Identity* (pp. 70–81). London: Sage.

GIBBS, J. C., and SCHNELL, S. V. (1985). 'Moral development "versus" socialization', *American Psychologist*, 40, 1071–80.

GORDON, C. (1968), 'Self-conceptions: configurations of content', in C. Gordon and K. J. Gergen (eds.), *The Self in Social Interaction* (pp. 115–36). New York: Wiley and Sons.

GORDON, C., and GERGEN, K. J. (1968), 'The nature and dimensions of self: introduction', in C. Gordon and K. J. Gergen (eds.), *The Self in Social Interaction* (pp. 33–39). New York: Wiley.

GUDYKUNST, W. B. (1988), 'Culture and intergroup processes', in M. H. Bond (ed.), *The Cross-Cultural Challenge to Social Psychology* (pp. 165–81). London: Sage.

HALLOWELL, A. I. (1976), *Contributions to Anthropology: selected papers of A. I. Hallowell*. Chicago: University of Chicago Press.

HARDMAN, C. (1981), 'The psychology of conformity and self-expression among the Lohorung Rai of East Nepal', in P. Heelas and A. Lock (eds.), *Indigenous Psychologies: the anthropology of the self* (pp. 161–80). London: Academic Press.

HARRÉ, R. (1981), 'Psychological variety', in P. Heelas and A. Lock (eds.), *Indigenous Psychologies: the anthropology of the self* (pp. 79–103). London: Academic Press.

HARRÉ, R. (1989), 'Language games and texts of identity', in J. Shotter and K. J. Gergen (eds.), *Text of Identity* (pp. 20–35). London: Sage.

HEELAS, P., and LOCK, A. (eds.) (1981), *Indigenous Psychologies: the anthropology of the self*. London: Academic Press.

HERMANS, H. J. M., KEMPEN, H. J. G., and VAN LOON, R. J. P. (in press), 'The dialogical self: beyond individualism and rationalism', *American Psychologist*.

HO, D. Y. F. (1985), 'Cultural values and professional issues in clinical psychology: implications from the Hong Kong experience', *American Psychologist*, 40, 1212–18.

HOFSTEDE, G. (1980), *Cultures Consequences: international differences in work-related values*. Beverly Hills: Sage.

HOGAN, R. (1975), 'Theoretical egocentrism and the problem of compliance', *American Psychologist*, 30, 533–40.

HOLDSTOCK, T. L. (1987), *Education for a New Nation*. Johannesburg: Africa Transpersonal Association.

HOLDSTOCK, T. L. (1990a), 'Can client-centered therapy transcend its monocultural roots?', in G. Lietaer, J. Rombauts, and R. van Balen (eds.), *Client-Centered and Experiential Psychotherapy in the Nineties* (pp. 109–21). Leuven: Leuven University Press.

HOLDSTOCK, T. L. (1990b, August), 'The self-concept since James: from "I" and "Me" towards "We".' Paper presented at the 1990 Principles Congress, Amsterdam.

HOLDSTOCK, T. L. (1990c). 'Violence in schools: discipline', in B. McKendrick and W. Hoffmann (eds.), *People and Violence in South Africa* (pp. 341–72). Cape Town: Oxford University Press.

HOLDSTOCK, T. L. (1991), 'Bodily awareness: a neglected dimension in Western education', in E. H. Katzenellenbogen and J. R. Potgieter (eds.), *Sociological Perspectives of Human Movement Activity* (pp. 44–52). Stellenbosch: Stellenbosch University Press.

HOWELL, S. (1981), 'Rules not words', in P. Heelas and A. Lock (eds.), *Indigenous Psychologies: the anthropology of the self* (pp. 133–43). London: Academic Press.

HSU, F. L. K. (1985), 'The self in cross-cultural perspective', in A. J. Marsella, G. DeVos, and F. L. K. Hsu (eds.), *Culture and Self: Asian and Western perspectives* (pp. 24–55). London: Tavistock.

JAHODA, G. (1988), 'J'accuse', in M. H. Bond (ed.), *The Cross-*

*Cultural Challenge to Social Psychology* (pp. 86–95). London: Sage.

JAMES, W. (1890/1950), *Principles of Psychology*. Cambridge, Ma: Harvard University Press.

JAMES, W. (1892), *Psychology: briefer course*. London: Macmillan.

JOHNSON, F. (1985), 'The Western concept of self', in A. J. Marsella, G. DeVos, and F. L. K. Hsu (eds.), *Culture and Self: Asian and Western perspectives* (pp. 91–138). London: Tavistock.

JOSSELSON, R. (1987), *Finding Herself: pathways to identity development in women*. London: Jossey-Bass.

JOSSELSON, R. (1990, September), 'Identity and relatedness in the life cycle.' Paper presented at the symposium on Identity and Development, Amsterdam.

KELLY, G. (1955), *The Psychology of Personal Constructs*. New York: Norton.

KIMURA, B. (1971), 'Mitmenschlichkeit in der psychiatrie', *Zeitschrift für Klinische Psychologie und Psychotherapie, 19,* 3–13.

KLEINMAN, A. (1980), *Patients and Healers in the Context of Culture*. Berkeley: University of California Press.

KOJIMA, H. (1984), 'A significant stride toward the comparative study of control', *American Psychologist, 39,* 972–73.

LASZLO, E. (1972), *The Systems View of the World: the natural philosophy of the new developments in the sciences*. New York: Braziller.

LEWIN, K. (1951), *Field Theory in Social Science*. Chicago: University of Chicago Press.

MACINTYRE, A. (1988), *Whose Justice? Which Rationality?* Notre Dame: University of Notre Dame Press.

MALPASS, R. S. (1988), 'Why not cross-cultural psychology? A characterization of some mainstream views', in M. H. Bond (ed.), *The Cross-Cultural Challenge to Social Psychology* (pp. 29–35). London: Sage.

MARKUS, H., and WURF, E. (1987), 'The dynamic self-concept: a social psychological perspective', *Annual Review of Psychology, 38,* 299–337.

MEAD, G. H. (1968), 'The genesis of the self', in C. Gordon and K. J. Gergen (eds.), *The Self in Social Interaction* (pp. 51–59). New York: Wiley.

MILLER, J. G. (1988), 'Bridging the content-structure dichotomy: culture and the self', in M. H. Bond (ed.), *The Cross-Cultural Challenge to Social Psychology* (pp. 266–81). London: Sage.

PERLOFF, R. (1987), 'Self-interest and personal responsibility redux', *American Psychologist*, 42, 3–11.

PRIBRAM, K. (In press), *Brain and Perception: holonomy and structure in figural processing*.

PRIGOGINE, I., and STENGERS, I. (1984), *Order out of Chaos: man's new dialogue with nature*. Boulder, Co: Shambhala.

PRILLELTENSKY, I. (1989), 'Psychology and the status quo', *American Psychologist*, 44, 795–802.

ROGERS, C. R. (1959), 'A theory of therapy, personality and interpersonal relationships as developed in the client-centered framework', in S. Koch (ed.), *Psychology: a study of science*, Vol. 3, *Formulations of the person and the social context* (pp. 184–256). New York: McGraw-Hill.

ROGERS, C. R. (1977), *Carl Rogers on Personal Power: inner strength and its revolutionary impact*. New York: Delacorte Press.

ROTTER, J. B. (1954), *Social Learning and Clinical Psychology*. Englewood Cliffs, NJ: Prentice-Hall.

SAMPSON, E. E. (1985), 'The decentralization of identity: toward a revised concept of personal and social order', *American Psychologist*, 40, 1203–11.

SAMPSON, E. E. (1988), 'The debate on individualism: indigenous psychologies of the individual and their role in personal and societal functioning', *American Psychologist*, 43, 15–22.

SAMPSON, E. E. (1989a), 'The challenge of social change for psychology: globalization and psychology's theory of the person', *American Psychologist*, 44, 914–21.

SAMPSON, E. E. (1989b), 'The deconstruction of the self', in J. Shotter and K. J. Gergen (eds.), *Texts of Identity* (pp. 1–19). London: Sage.

SARASON, S. B. (1981), 'An asocial psychology and a misdirected clinical psychology', *American Psychologist*, 36, 827–36.

SCHWARTZ, B. (1986), *The Battle for Human Nature. Science, morality and modern life.* New York: Norton.

SCHWEDER, R. A., and BOURNE, E. J. (1989), 'Does the concept of the person vary cross-culturally?' in A. J. Marsella and G. M. White (eds.), *Cultural Conceptions of Mental Health and Therapy* (pp. 97–137). London: D. Reidel.

SINHA, J. B. P. (1984), 'Towards partnership for relevant research in the third world', *International Journal of Psychology*, 19, 169–77.

SLUGOSKI, B. R., and GINSBURG, G. P. (1989), 'Ego identity and explanatory speech', in J. Shotter and K. J. Gergen (eds.), *Texts of Identity* (pp. 36–55). London: Sage.

SMITH, J. (1981), 'Self and experience in Maori culture', in P. Heelas and A. Lock (eds.), *Indigenous Psychologies: the anthropology of the self* (pp. 145–59). London: Academic Press.

SMUTS, J. C. (1926), *Holism and Evolution.* London: Macmillan.

SPENCE, J. T. (1985), 'Achievement American style: the rewards and costs of individualism', *American Psychologist*, 40, 1285–95.

TEDESCHI, J. T. (1988), 'How does one describe a platypus? An outsider's questions for cross-cultural psychology', in M. H. Bond (ed.), *The Cross-Cultural Challenge to Social Psychology* (pp. 14–28). London: Sage.

TRIANDIS, H. C. (1988), 'Cross-cultural contributions to theory in social psychology', in M. H. Bond (ed.), *The Cross-Cultural Challenge to Social Psychology* (pp. 122–40). London: Sage.

TUAN, YI-FU (1982), *Segmented Words and Self.* Minneapolis: University of Minnesota Press.

VAN DER VEER, R. (1985), 'Similarities between the theories of G. H. Mead and L. S. Vygotskij: an explanation?' in S. Bem, H. van Rappard, and W. van Hoorn (eds.), *Studies in the History of Psychology and Social Sciences*, Vol. 3. Leiden: Psychologisch Instituut.

VON BERTALANFFY, L. (1969), *General Systems Theory: foundations, development, applications.* New York: Braziller.

WATERMAN, A. S. (1981), 'Individualism and interdependence', *American Psychologist*, 36, 762–73.

WEI-MING, T. (1985), 'Selfhood and otherness in Confucian thought', in A. J. Marsella, G. DeVos, and F. L. K. Hsu (eds.), *Culture and Self: Asian and Western perspectives* (pp. 231–51). London: Tavistock.

WEXLER, D. A. (1974), 'A cognitive theory of experiencing, self-actualization, and therapeutic process', in D. A. Wexler and L. N. Rice (eds.), *Innovations in Client-Centered Therapy* (pp. 49–116). New York: Wiley.

WILBER, K. (ed.) (1982), *The Holographic Paradigm and other Paradoxes: exploring the leading edge of science*. London: Shambala.

WILBER, K. (ed.) (1984), *Quantum Questions: mystical writings of the world's great physicists*. London: Shambala.

YANG, K. S. (1988), 'Will societal modernization eventually eliminate cross-cultural psychological differences?' in M. H. Bond (ed.), *The Cross-Cultural Challenge to Social Psychology* (pp. 67–85). London: Sage.

YOUNG, L. B. (1986), *The Unfinished Universe*. New York: Simon and Schuster.

# From Rogers to Gleick and Back Again

## RUTH SANFORD

### THE THEORY OF THE PERSON-CENTRED APPROACH AND THE THEORY OF CHAOS

This chapter is a reflection upon the parallels between the theory of the person-centred approach and the theory of chaos. A landmark in the latter was the publication in 1987 of Robert Gleick's book *Chaos: making a new science*. After eighteen years of studying the theory which underlies the structure of the person-centred approach, I find that Rogers' descriptions of a new way of being and of the process of becoming, move alongside the new way of thinking described by Gleick in his book on chaos. To quote from Gleick's prologue: 'Chaos is a science of process rather than state, of becoming rather than being' (p. 5).

After experiencing the application of person-centred theory in the therapeutic one-to-one relationship as well as in intensive groups, training programmes, university classes and intimate day-to-day relationships, I find strong evidence that the theory has a solid scientific base. My focus, therefore, is on Carl Rogers the scientist who, as the theory of chaos unfolds, is clearly in the vanguard of this new science.

## PROCESS

'Chaos is a science of process.' That is the first important point to hold on to because, as I see it, process is a word which indicates one of the parallels between the new science and the new way of being which Rogers evolved and which he practised.

In 1961, Rogers, in *On Becoming a Person*, devoted a chapter to 'A Process Conception of Psychotherapy'. In his later works, he speaks of empathy or deep empathic listening, not as a state but as a process that works quietly and dynamically.

I have spoken of the parallel that is expressed in the word 'process'. I shall now speak of some of the many other ways in which Carl Rogers' work, I believe, parallels the new science, not necessarily in the chronological order in which they have evolved.

## UNIVERSALITY

I was reminded recently that universality has different meanings in the popular vernacular and in science. Nevertheless, I shall use the term and try to define it in its various uses.

Rogers addressed universality with two somewhat different meanings himself. One is embraced in his saying, 'The more personal is the more general.' I have found that if I speak very deeply from my own experience and my own open heart, what I have to say will speak to the hearts of many people in many countries from many backgrounds.

In my experience the more personal is the more general. An example that comes quickly to mind is the one-page piece first written as one of my weekly columns in the local newspaper under the by-line, 'As I See It'. The title of the piece was 'Loving with an Open Hand'. It was a distillation of more than thirty years of my life. It came about at a point in my life when I called a friend and said, 'My life is getting so tangled; it's like a tangled piece of yarn. If I could only get hold of one end of it I think I could unravel it but I can't find that end.'

My husband was ill. My daughter was small. The two mothers had come to be with us to help and I was trying to be a good wife, a good mother, a good daughter-in-law, a good daughter, and in the process found that I was taking responsibility for members of the family and was losing myself. I was simply going under. This very good friend helped me to see that others in the family had their own strengths and that if I let them use their own strengths they would become stronger, that I was not responsible for everyone. In one week of very intensive work, I came to that realization.

Waking up from a nap one afternoon, the words came to me very clearly: 'You've been protective. What does protective mean? It means I protect what I possess.' I was horrified.

The change that I made there, I believe strongly, made a difference to the whole future of my family. I used in 'Loving with an Open Hand' the metaphor of a butterfly coming out of a cocoon; a very helpful person who wanted to help the butterfly come out of the cocoon loosened the thread. The butterfly came out but had such weak wings it could never fly. I find that wherever I have gone in the world – South Africa, the Soviet Union, Mexico – someone has spoken to me and said. 'Oh! You wrote "Loving with an Open Hand". I have it up on my refrigerator door [or I have it by my bedside]. It has spoken to me.'

So, that the more personal is the more general has very real meaning for me, and there is a universality of the human condition, the human experience. In South Africa, England, France, Mexico – almost every class or group with which I've spoken – I've had this feedback.

In *A Way of Being* (1980, p. 114), Rogers said one of the bases for his theory is the self-actualizing tendency which is at work in individual organisms including the human organism. The universality of this tendency as expressed in other forms of life extends to the universe itself and is called the formative tendency. This is what Rogers said in *A Way of Being* about the formative tendency:

We are tapping into a tendency which permeates all of organic life – a tendency to become all the complexity of which the organism is capable. And on an even larger scale, I believe we are tuning in to a potent creative tendency which has formed our universe, from the smallest snowflake to the largest galaxy, from the lowly amoeba to the most sensitive and gifted of persons. And perhaps we are touching the cutting edge of our ability to transcend ourselves, to create new and more spiritual directions in human evolution. This kind of formulation for me is a philosophical base for the person-centered approach. (p. 134.)

In 1951, in his *Client-Centered Therapy*, he made reference to the self-actualizing tendency, although at that time he did not use the term. It grew out of his rejection of certain concepts common in therapy at the time: the regressive tendency, the death instinct, disruptive forces, the closed systems of classical science and the closed system of the science or the practice of therapy.

## FROM CLOSED SYSTEMS TO OPEN SYSTEMS

It is important to note that what Rogers was questioning was the established and the classical forms of psychotherapy, the analytical and the behavioural approaches which had been widely accepted. When he put his trust in the open system, the self-actualizing tendency, and genuinely believed that that system was at work within each individual, he could no longer function within a closed system. What he was doing was the same thing that the new scientists have done in putting aside the classical science which is built on predictable structures. Rogers was basing his approach to therapy on his experience.

'My recent thinking', he wrote in 1951, 'tends more and more toward the individual as an organism with a rather definite need for structure and with almost unlimited potential provided the environment gives him the opportunity to become aware of his needs and of his wells of positive expressivity' (p. 167), which again defines for Rogers the role of the therapist as being quite different from the role which had been defined previously.

He was defining somewhat tentatively at that point the self-actualizing tendency. 'The self-actualizing tendency', he wrote later in 1980 in *A Way of Being* (p. 115), 'is characteristic of organic life of which the human organism is one. Individuals have within themselves vast resources for altering their self-concepts, their basic attitudes and self-directed behavior. These resources can be tapped if a definable climate of known facilitative, psychological attitudes can be provided.'

He later defined the conditions as being:

1. Deep empathic listening.
2. Unconditional positive regard or acceptance of the other person and the other person's reality.
3. Genuineness or realness – not having to hide behind a professional front or a desk or a white coat or other device.

In *On Personal Power* (1977, p. 8), Rogers made an even stronger statement which he did not repeat in this 1980 definition. 'This tendency', he said, referring to the self-actualizing tendency, 'can be thwarted but cannot be destroyed without destroying the whole organism.'

This leads to a little story about Rogers. As a small boy he lived on a farm. The potatoes were put in the basement to keep over the winter and he noticed that towards spring many of those potatoes became small, dried up and wizened, but that they sent out little delicate white shoots which found their way toward the only light in that dark basement, a cellar window high up.

This illustration he carried through his life as an example of the self-actualizing tendency. These fragile shoots would never become the strong potato plants which they were meant to be. They could never produce other potatoes but they were doing the best they could in the environment which they had – stunted but still trying.

Ilya Prigogine, to whom he referred frequently, the Belgian scientist and philosopher who received the Nobel prize in chemistry the same year that *On Personal Power* was published, speaks of an open system. He said what Rogers said but in a different language.

Coming from the discipline of statistical and chemical physics, he was open to his experience even as Rogers was open to his. He used his own terminology to describe 'the spectrum that runs from simple, self-organizing systems, to the whirlpool and Jupiter's Red Spot, to more complicated, dissipative structures and finally to highly complex, self-actualizing, autopoetic or self-making systems such as ourselves, the human being.'

Open systems are those that depend on interaction with their environment, the larger world. According to the theory of open systems, an organism in either a state of order or of chaos by the incidence of perturbations or fluctuations is thereby given a choice, a choice of bifurcation (bifurcation being a point of branching) a choice of moving from order (any of these directions are possible when a branching or a choice takes place) to chaos or from chaos toward order or remaining in chaos or order of a greater or lesser degree, but when turbulence or perturbations are introduced into a *self-organizing* organism in an open system, change will take place.

That is Prigogine's concept. Now I hear Rogers and Prigogine saying in different terminology that the human organism, which Rogers referred to as the individual, is an open system, self-organizing, self-actualizing, which means what its life depends on the flow between the self and its environment which cannot remain in equilibrium if the organism is to stay alive but is, rather, in a constant interchange of energy.

If one accepts the concept of an open system, which Rogers and Prigogine both do, then the organism is nudged at this point from the condition of entropy or the tendency toward death by means of perturbations, large or small, which permit the organism to export the excess entropy.* The self-actualizing tendency is at work within the organism with a movement toward another form or another level of organization.

Rogers says 'toward greater complexity' (1980, p. 133). Prigo-

---

* Davies, Paul, in *The New Physics* (p. 5), Cambridge: Cambridge University Press, 1989.

gine says 'of increasing complexity' (1984, p. 12). Prigogine implies but does not state that this tendency exists in the self-organizing organism as long as the organism exists. He simply says it is. Rogers says, 'It persists.'

Philosophers, theologians, and logicians may see this parallel in different lights but my light leads me to put it this way: Prigogine says that an open system, when perturbations occur, tends to export entropy and to move in the direction of greater complexity. The tendency exists in the organism. It is.

Rogers says that it not only exists in the human organism but it persists in the face of destructive forces in the environment and can be destroyed only by destroying the organism itself. In his later years, Rogers expressed the belief that this tendency toward greater complexity does not rule out transformation to another form of existence.

## IRREVERSIBILITY

Another point at which Rogers and Prigogine meet is captured in the word 'irreversibility'. This for Prigogine involves the concept of time.

As a layman I shall not attempt to penetrate the core of the issue of time which is so profound that it occupied many years of the life and thought of Albert Einstein.

Gleick says, 'Relativity eliminated the Newtonian illusion of absolute space and time; quantum theory eliminated the Newtonian dream of a controllable measurement process; chaos eliminates the Laplacian fantasy of deterministic predictability' (1987, p. 6).

Heraclitus expressed the idea, congenial to Taoism, that one can never step into the same river twice, meaning that minute by minute the river changes as it flows and, although it is the same river, it is never the same in any two consecutive moments or days or weeks or years.

As I become more and more aware of my body and of my feelings I know that I am not and can never be exactly the same as I was an hour previously. Interactions within myself, with the part of the world immediately surrounding me and the persons with whom I have interacted have already brought about some change.

The forward thrust toward increased complexity in all open systems is irregular but persistent in its movement. Carl Rogers' experience of irreversibility as drawn from various statements and writings can be paraphrased as: The individual once engaged in the process of change and growth, once gaining a new insight, cannot return to yesterday's being. That organism is forever changed in some way.

The concept of irreversibility then is inherent in the self-actualizing tendency. The self-actualizing tendency in the larger environment, which leads again directly to the formative tendency in the universe, means that we are not alone and this to me has a great significance. As a human being, I am not alone in this thrust forward toward greater complexity. It means that we are not alone in the forward thrust, whether it be from order or from chaos; we may go from order to chaos or chaos to order and not even be aware of the perturbations that have brought it about.

## LISTENING

A further point which Rogers and Prigogine have in common as I see it is listening, which brings us to the question of communication. Prigogine said that communication within the organism and between the organism and its environment is essential to the life of that organism.

In reaching this point Rogers was far, far ahead. The first chapter of *A Way of Being* is called 'Communication'; the first aspect of communication which he addresses in that chapter is listening. He speaks of the enjoyment he feels:

When I can really hear someone it puts me in touch with him; it enriches my life. It is through hearing people that I have learned all that I know about individuals, about personality, about interpersonal relationships. There is another peculiar satisfaction in really hearing someone: It is like listening to the music of the spheres because beyond the immediate message of the person, no matter what that might be, there is the universal. Hidden in all personal communications which I really hear there seem to be orderly psychological laws, aspects of the same order we find in the universe as a whole. (1980. p. 8.)

He raised the question – and he raised this every time he had an interview or was meeting with a group – 'Can I hear the sound, the sense and the shape of this person's inner world? Is it going to be possible for me to do that and to stay with it? Can I resonate to what he is saying so deeply that I sense the meaning he is afraid to express as well as what he is saying?' (Rogers, 1980, p. 8).

An illustration of such listening makes the meaning very clear, I believe. Rogers recounted his experience of meeting a young man who tried to say why he was consulting Rogers. Did he have a purpose? Was there something he wanted? What was he asking Rogers for? He said, I don't know. There's nothing in this world I want.

Rogers accepted his statement at face value and as they went along with the conversation the young man finally said, there is something I want to say. I want to live. That is, I want to keep on living.

At that point, Rogers sensed that beneath the words perhaps the young man was saying that there was a time when he didn't want to live. As they talked further the young man spoke of a recent suicide attempt. That was deep listening.

In such a relationship Rogers talked little and had time to resonate to the other, to be in communication, to trust his own experience of that communication, was open to the other, to himself and to his intuitive knowing. We have spoken of listening as a kind of resonance.

## RESONANCE IN GROUPS AND IN SCIENTIFIC MODELS

Turning to the field of dynamics, non-linear oscillators can also be a good parallel for resonance in groups of persons and organizations. Facilitators of groups working within the person-centred model frequently experience the building up of resonance within a group so intense that it becomes unbearable to one or more of the participants. At that point in a group, when the resonance becomes so strong, a person may tell a joke, break the tension, break the strength of the resonance. Other persons may get up and leave the room.

Rogers was aware of this: he spoke of the wisdom of the group and the movement of the group and the trust and the self-actualizing tendency within the group even when it was lost in chaos.

The non-linear oscillators demonstrate that the force introduced by resonance can be so great as to change the system to a new resonance or to a new chaos. This parallel between non-linear oscillators and the building of resonance between individuals in a person-centred group would be highly improbable in a system that is not open, in other words, in a closed authoritarian group. At the base of the open system in groups is the self-actualizing tendency of the individuals within the group.

What is the parallel in the new science? James Gleick opens his book on chaos with a quotation from John Updike, a couplet:

> Human was the music
> Natural was the static.

In these two lines is the clue to the relationship between Rogers' listening and the new science. It is the awareness of ears that had been tuned to the beautiful ordered sounds of music created by human beings. I think the parallel is with pre-structured, well-organized systems of psychotherapy from which Rogers came, created by human beings, and the intrusion of static, the disruptive, the unexpected, the unintended sounds or noise that interfere with the pursuit of the orderly beauty of a created structure. The static for the therapist can be the individual, the unexpected, the sometimes unintelligible attempts a client makes to express deep feelings.


## 'LISTENING TO THE NOISE': ROGERS AND THE NEW SCIENTISTS

Herein lies the existing story of making a new science as Gleick tells it – a new way of thinking. It has first of all to do with the various disciplines within the new sciences and the hard sciences. It involved mathematicians, physicists, applied physicists, chemists, biologists, astronomers, economists rather than the borderline or not so pure scientists, the sociologists, the anthropologists, the psychologists and so on.

I have learned that there was a hierarchy between pure sciences and the applied sciences. The pure scientist did not talk very well with the applied scientist because it seemed one was just a cut above the other. There was very little communication or recognition between the two. Placing the term 'applied' before the designated discipline was a kind of stigma.

The startling development in recent years is the slow and grudging acknowledgement among pure scientists that what they had long considered noise or error when they were working on these beautiful equations of theirs, was significant. They would run an equation, replicate it on a computer, and after a while somehow the orderliness began to fade out, disappear, and a lot of seemingly irrelevant information was being fed in. Suddenly the whole orderly progression went berserk.

They assumed that something was wrong with the computer; something was wrong with the equation; or something was wrong with their calculations. They would put it aside with, 'Well, this is a mistake. We'll start over.' They were not listening to what the noise said. Then, here and there, scientists began to say, 'I wonder if there is some meaning in that noise. I wonder if it's worth listening to.'

As Gleick refers to it, there was a succession of such scientists. I shall mention only one or two by way of illustration. They may not be the most prominent or the most important but these pioneers were courageous, curious, open-minded, adventurous individuals, were willing to listen to their intuition as well as to follow their equations and their technical knowledge, struggle day by day and night by night to uncover what these unpredictable incursions might mean; what they might be saying to someone who could be listening with an open mind. That was the beginning of the process of listening to that which had very little meaning in the classical history of science and mathematics.

Like Leonardo da Vinci and his flying machine, their endeavours were presented with insurmountable barriers of time. How long would it take to run these equations out to millions of iterations? It would take a man's lifetime. Space, time and materials were inadequate. Some new invention was needed before ideas could be translated rapidly enough into tangible, visible form, before predictability or unpredictability could be tested – predictability or randomness, order or chaos.

The emergence of the high-powered computer introduced a whole new dimension, opened up almost infinite possibilities for exploration of predictability and randomness as they affect organisms and the universe itself.

Gleick tells the story of Mitchell Feigenbaum who, among many others, led the way in this exploration. He was one of a group of Los Alamos scientists who was known for solving other people's problems, doing a lot of thinking, trying out all kinds of time sequences for himself, staying up all night trying to live days of varying numbers of hours, seemingly getting nowhere but doing a lot of thinking and beginning intuitively to get the sense that he was on to something deep. He did not know what but he was listening to his intuition.

Feigenbaum discovered a number, the Feigenbaum number, that is universal, i.e. the same for all curves which have a single, maximum value. He was studying simple numerical functions but he believed that his theory expressed a natural law about systems, something in mathematics, physics, biology and the point of transition between orderly and turbulent. He did what most mathematicians and scientists had shunned.

Although an intuitive knowing had produced no hard proof, he persisted. He wrote papers even when he had no hard proof and submitted them for publication. He persisted in the face of repeated rejections. One editor rejected a paper of his for publication because 'It is not suitable to the reading audience of the journal.'

Many years later that editor acknowledged Feigenbaum had opened up a whole new field of science but he still persisted in saying, 'I was right. I was right to reject that publication because it was not appropriate to that audience' (Gleick, 1987, p. 181).

Rogers found himself in a similar kind of situation at the beginning of his professional career. He was not accepted by psychiatrists as a therapist; he was not accepted even in psychology departments as a psychologist; he was not in the mainstream. He turned to psychiatric social workers; rose to a prominent organizational position there; then, recognized by the American Association for Applied Psychology, was invited to become a professor in the Sociology and Education Department and finally, at the University of Rochester, was invited by the Department of Psychology to offer courses in that department.

Fortunately Feigenbaum also persisted. This was a point at which a real explosion began to take place in the whole concept of listening to noise and this field of new science. The scientists began listening not only to noise but to their own intuition and to its meaning.

In 1979, Feigenbaum went to a conference in Corsica where he met Michael Barnsley, an Oxford-educated, English mathematician. 'That', said Gleick, 'is where Barnsley first learned about universality and period doubling and infinite cascades of bifurcations' (1987, p. 215) in a system or organism.

Barnsley began to ask questions about Feigenbaum's sequences, cycles of two, four, eight, sixteen. 'Did they appear by magic out of a mathematical void or did they suggest a shadow of something deeper still? Barnsley's intuition was that they must be part of some fabulous fractal object so far hidden from view' (Gleick, 1987, p. 215).

He wrote a paper and sent it off to *Communications in Mathematical Physics* for publication. The editor, David Ruelle, recognized that he had rediscovered a buried piece of work written by Gaston Julia, a French mathematician, fifty years before. This is what is important. He sent Barnsley a message, 'Get in touch with Mandelbrot' (Gleick, 1987, p. 216). Mandelbrot is known as the father of fractals who opened up a new and visual world to the new scientists.

There was so much vitality. They were crossing the barriers that had separated them before. They were becoming parts of open systems. They were hastening to get their ideas out, to communicate them, and the old barrier of one not speaking to the other, one not working with the other, feeling that one was a cut above the other, was breaking down. In the breaking down of that old form, Gleick says – and I think this is very significant in terms of Rogers' work – 'Where chaos begins, classical science stops' (1987, p. 3). Here, again, was an openness, a listening to experience, a moving on into the unknown which could be very frightening.

## FRACTALS

Fractals become more real by way of visual presentation of the fantastically beautiful plates from *The Beauty of Fractals* by H. O. Peitgen and P. Richter (1986). These illustrations show some of the wonders of the modern computer that have made possible an exploration of the information provided by noise, made possible a new way of thinking, a new way of science. We see in fractals, made visible and possible by high-powered computers, the non-linear, irregular, complex and beautiful patterns that contrast strongly with the linear, regular, simple, symmetrical forms of the classical, mechanical, original Newtonian science. Very simply, these coloured forms are created by assigning a colour to a given value in an equation which is iterated many, many times. At this point

I would like to move back to the question of open systems and their application in psychology.

## RETURN TO OPEN SYSTEMS: PSYCHOLOGY

An organism can be an amoeba, a single cell; it can be a human being; it can be a termite colony; it can be Jupiter's Red Spot; it can be a human organization; it can be a family; it can be, in the beginning, a fractured group in conflict. I shall go step by step through some of our experiences in groups. The following patterns appear in different groups all over the world but a similar progression seems to occur somewhere in the process each time.

As Rogers and I worked with groups of all sizes from 25 to 2,000 in Mexico, Hungary, South Africa, the Soviet Union, England, Kenya, Austria, Zimbabwe, Ireland and the United States, we learned more and more to trust the process in intensive groups. This is the key word that Rogers kept using – trusting the process, i.e. the process involved in the self-actualizing tendency.

Rogers referred to it as 'the wisdom of the group' (1980, p. 196). He experienced the same process when he was at work in Japan and Brazil and other countries, all of which seems to indicate that this wisdom of the organism is evident in varying cultures.

Initially, in the interest of clarity I made references to steps in the group process and I tried to number the steps but repeatedly lost count. I asked myself the question, 'Why am I having so much difficulty enumerating steps in the process – sometimes six, sometimes eight, but never the same count twice?' My answer was that I was trying to build a step structure to express a fluid process. I now feel ready to look again at the group process in an open system.

Groups usually assemble with expectations of a more or less orderly way of proceeding. As long as there is communication, even if it is at a somewhat casual, shallow level, it continues to be more or less orderly and polite but by the very nature of person-centredness, it is functioning in a non-linear way. Many dimensions are involved because every person in this kind of group is free to become a potential perturbation to introduce his or her own kind of turbulence. The organism is not held to a single line by some rule or authoritarian person or by a ready-made structure.

By the action of one person, a small perturbation is introduced into this open system. There is a choice of behaviours within the organization: a bifurcation or a branching, the possibility of new choices. The organization becomes thereby much more complex.

Then other individuals introduce their choices. There are many bursts of energy in many different directions. Each person is in a potential leadership role. That's empowerment of an individual within a group. Each one can become a leader.

The organism becomes even more complex. There are more bifurcations, more dimensions. It seems that it's going to fly apart. It's in a state of chaos. Rogers referred to it sometimes as chaos when he wondered if struggling through it for two or three days in a workshop was worth the pain and the effort, but he always came back to the longer view. The term which he used, particularly in the Soviet Union, was patience, patience to trust the process, to trust the self-actualizing tendency and to live through the pain and the disorder of chaos.

In a group in Moscow in 1986, we experienced this kind of chaos during a full day. Participants in the group implored us, 'Do something about this chaos or it will go on for days! What are you here for anyway? You are doing nothing!' and 'We'll never get anywhere!' Toward the close of that day we asked that the group sit quietly for a few moments before we went home. The next day people came back with a very different sense of why they were there. We trusted that they would find their own way and that it would mean a lot more to them than our finding it for them or trying to point it out.

A similar experience has been repeated many times in workshops. Perhaps there will be a time when trusting the process does not work but I have not yet seen it.

If a group is functioning as an open system, individual organisms within that group become aware of communication within themselves, and of communication with others within the group, both of which are essential to the coming together of that group as a community. The process has translated into human action what Prigogine defined as essential to the continuing life of an organism.

As the group continues in their process within the functioning philosophy of the person-centred approach, someone in the group iterates the concept of communication. Someone says, 'We are not listening to one another. I want to hear you.' In fact, in the Soviet Union the only kind of facilitation that Rogers and I used during those first couple of days was to say, 'Wait a minute. I didn't hear what you said and I really want to hear.' For a short time then there was some listening. In a group somewhere, a facilitator probably – or possibly one of the participants – will say, 'Wait a minute. Things are going too fast. I want to hear you,' and communication is re-established. Prigogine is also saying that communication must be there in order for that organism to exist, to continue living.

When listening does take place and someone begins to listen at this point of awareness, the group is thrown into another kind of diversity, a diversity that includes a new sense of respect for the other person, which is one of Rogers' three conditions. More specifically it means listening to the other person, having respect for that person's point of view whether or not it agrees with mine, saying 'Your reality is different from mine and I may not like it but I accept that your reality is just as real for you as mine is for me and therefore, I want to give you space. I want to hear you.'

Then follows an increased sense of awareness within oneself of what is going on which Rogers called congruence or realness, being aware of the feelings that are flowing in me at the time and being able to communicate them to someone else.

For example, in the 1975 workshop at Mills College, Ann, a participant, called the group back. In a quiet, insistent voice she spoke up and said, 'Back here Vincente told about his pain and the suffering he was feeling for his people and we didn't hear him and he sat down unheard. I want to go back to Vincente' (1977, p. 146).

Rogers said that it turned a whole workshop around. Because of her intervention, everyone who had been striving to express their own passionate feelings about their own doings, striving to be heard

269

rather than listening, paused. He called it the beginning of community, a point which usually does not come about until after chaos has set in in a group.

Chaos, as anyone who has been through it knows, is very painful but can also be very creative. After the chaos came the turning point. Rogers wrote later that he went back to his room after the experience feeling pride and awe at being present at the birth pangs of something new in this world, at the beginning of community. Each time a group of disparate, non-engaged, perhaps openly hostile persons finds their way through to a sense of genuine involvement in the hopes, the pains or joys of one another, it is a fresh and awesome experience.

The new scientist would say that it is the order that can come out of chaos when turbulence or perturbations are introduced. The scientist speaking in the person-centred mode would say order can come out of chaos if certain, definable psychological conditions exist. In this situation it was deep empathic listening first, respect for the reality of others as well as for one's own reality, and being genuine.

Empowerment develops within the group and empowerment within the group itself took place again and again as we worked. We became aware that with every new group we were testing the hypothesis: You can trust the process of becoming, the wisdom of the group.

Gleick saw what I've just been talking about. There's a point where classical science ends and the new science begins, where process replaces a state in our vocabulary, where we trust in the process in individuals or in a group.

Carl Rogers, the scientist* and visionary, expresses his hope for

---

* Howard Kirschenbaum and Valerie Henderson (1989, p. 201) call attention to Rogers' contributions to scientific research in psychology: 'Psychological theory and particularly research occupied a central focus for the first thirty-five years of Rogers' career.' Kirschenbaum, in his biography of Carl Rogers (1979, p. 394), says, '[He was] the first psychologist in history to receive both the APA's Scientific Contribution Award and their distinguished Professional Contribution Award.' The citation for the first of these awards recognized him '. . . for developing an original method to objectify the description and analysis of the psychotherapeutic process,

the development of psychology as embracing and practising a more human science of the person in the concluding paragraphs of the chapter 'New Challenges to Helping Professions' in *A Way of Being*. He speaks of the possibility of the profession of psychology or the science of psychology becoming a self-actualizing organism.

> I have raised the question of whether psychology will remain a narrow technological fragment of a science, tied to an outdated philosophical conception of itself, clinging to a security blanket of observable behavior only; or whether it can possibly become a truly broad and creative science, rooted in a subjective vision, open to all aspects of the human condition, worthy of the name of a mature science.
>
> I have raised the question of whether we dare to turn from being a past-oriented remedial technology to focusing on future-oriented planning, taking our part in a chaotic world to build the environment where human beings can choose to learn, where minorities can choose to remake the establishment through relating to it, where people can learn to live cooperatively together . . .
>
> Each issue, in a word, represents for psychology a step towards self-actualization. If my perceptions have been even approximately correct, then the final question I would leave with you is, do we dare? (1980, pp. 257–58)

One of the things I heard Rogers say often was, 'This way of being is not for the faint-hearted and this process will never stop as long as there is life in us.'

If the open system then exists, which I choose to believe, the self-actualizing tendency does live in each of us. It is at work. Because we are self-actualizing, self-organizing, we can help to create that environment for others. We can move on closer and closer to our own potential. The process is irreversible. It is the

for formulating a testable theory of psychotherapy and its effects on personality and behavior, and for extensive systematic research to exhibit the value of the method and explore and test the implications of the theory . . .' (1989, p. 201).

directional pull if we can listen to it in ourselves and trust it in others.

I find also that Rogers was in the vanguard of this whole movement in the new science by so long ago discovering for himself, through his experience and through his listening, that these forces have worked and are working in psychology.

I firmly believe that there is a parallel between the basis of the person-centred theory, that is, the self-actualizing tendency and the formative tendency, and the new science of which chaos is a part. The difficult transition as I see it is between recognition of this intersection intellectually and acceptance of it in personal experience.

I wish to acknowledge with thanks Ed Bodfish and Cheryl Desrosiers for making this revision possible.

REFERENCES

BRIGGS, JOHN, and PEAT, F. DAVID (1989), *Turbulent Mirror: an illustrated guide to chaos theory and the science of wholeness.* New York: Harper and Row.

CAPRA, FRITJOF (1984), *The Tao of Physics.* New York: Bantam Books.

GLEICK, JAMES (1987), *Chaos: making of a new science.* New York: Viking Penguin.

KIRSCHENBAUM, HOWARD (1979), *On Becoming Carl Rogers.* New York: Delacorte Press.

KIRSCHENBAUM, HOWARD, and HENDERSON, VALERIE (1989), *The Carl Rogers Reader.* Boston: Houghton Mifflin.

PRIGOGINE, I., and STENGERS, I. (1984), *Order Out of Chaos: man's new dialogue with nature.* Boulder: Shambhala Publications.

ROGERS, CARL (1951), *Client-Centered Therapy.* Boston: Houghton Mifflin.

ROGERS, CARL (1961), *On Becoming a Person*. Boston: Houghton Mifflin.

ROGERS, CARL (1977), *Carl Rogers on Personal Power*. New York: Delacorte Press.

ROGERS, CARL (1980), *A Way of Being*. Boston: Houghton Mifflin.

ROGERS, CARL (1985), 'Rogers, Kohut and Erickson: a personal perspective on some similarities and differences.' Conference on Evolution of the Psychotherapies. Phoenix, 1985.

SANFORD, RUTH (1978), 'Loving with an Open Hand', *Wantagh-Seaford Observer*.

## · 14 ·

# Eclecticism: An Identity Crisis for Person-Centred Therapists

## ROBERT HUTTERER

### INTRODUCTION

If the person-centred approach is to survive and prosper, it is important for person-centred therapists to attain a clear sense of confidence in their approach and their identity within it. My starting point for this final chapter, therefore, is my observation of and concern about the fact that therapists coming from person-centred training programmes and calling themselves 'person-centred' not infrequently go on to seek their identity and success in a more eclectic way of doing therapy and see advantages in integrating techniques from other approaches to the detriment of their person-centred principles. Some even report a critical attitude to the traditional approach or conclude that the 'necessary and sufficient' assumption (Rogers, 1957) does not work in therapeutic practice.

I am inclined to view the appeal of an eclectic approach as a crisis of identity for the therapist in which two interacting components play a part. These are, on the one hand, the strong anti-dogmatism of Rogers' approach and, on the other, the pressures exerted by the professional environment in which the therapist must operate. Both factors create problems in the development of a distinctly person-centred identity. My purpose here, therefore, is to briefly explore these two factors in the hope that this will challenge us to consider our approach more deeply.

## THE DILEMMA WITHIN THE APPROACH

Let us look more closely at the two factors just identified: firstly the dilemma which exists within the approach itself. This has two poles. The first pole may be called 'anti-dogmatism'. It includes the attempt to free theoretical thinking of rigid concepts, a positive regard for direct experience and advocacy of the value of each therapist developing a personal individual style. The opposite pole is the commitment to a set of values which constitute the core of the person-centred approach.

The tension between these two poles was, for Rogers himself, a source of creative impulses. He was comfortable with it, and this was not surprising in view of his general tolerance for contradictions. For many others, however, who feel close to the person-centred approach or who want to come close to it, this tension is a source of confusion.

### ANTI-DOGMATISM

The person-centred approach strongly advocates openness to new insights. This can be, and frequently is, misunderstood as licence to do anything. When it is taken this way, however, the person-centred basic assumptions are likely to get lost. The demand upon the therapist to be strongly committed to the basic assumptions while simultaneously remaining anti-dogmatic can certainly be a source of confusion and dilemma.

Rogers was anti-dogmatic. This anti-dogmatic view is central to the tradition of person-centred therapy and Rogers has always pointed it out in a very radical way. It is expressed in his numerous references to the dangers of institutionalization of person-centred psychotherapy, in his fear that the person-centred approach could develop into a rigid and self-sufficient school that is frozen more in defending its own position than developing itself.

His anti-dogmatism is further expressed in his openness to other schools. He pointed out, for instance, that techniques from other therapeutic schools can also present a communication channel for a person-centred approach (Rogers, 1957). When Rogers was asked how far he took this principle, he answered that he would rather help a psychologist or psychotherapist who prefers a directive and controlling form of therapy, to clarify his or her aims and meanings, than convince him or her of the person-centred position.

This anti-dogmatic attitude is also expressed in the sceptical principle which states: Do not follow any authority but have confidence in your own experiences and develop your own personal style. Rogers has thus turned against all those who blindly follow and imitate him, thereby ignoring their own strength, their own potential.

Finally, this anti-dogmatic attitude comes through very consistently in his position as psychotherapy researcher. As researcher Rogers was interested in an objectively effective therapy for the client. In favour of objectivity he did not seem willing to protect a person-centred system of thought. In his stubborn adherence to objectivity in this respect, he was even willing to risk the self-destruction of the person-centred theory. The significance of psychotherapy research, in Rogers' words, 'is that a growing body of objectively verified knowledge of psychotherapy will bring about the gradual demise of "schools" of psychotherapy, including this one'. And one paragraph later: 'Out of this [research] should grow an increasingly effective, and continually changing psychotherapy which will neither have nor need any specific label' (Rogers, 1961, p. 268).

Rogers' stressing of progress in psychotherapy research rested on the hope that 'there will be less and less emphasis upon dogmatic and purely theoretical formulations.' (Rogers, 1961, p. 268.)

COMMITMENT

On the other hand, all Rogers seemed to be interested in was to work out, in ever more detail and differentiation, his approach, the concept which he had initiated: to extend its areas of application, to clarify central concepts and protect them from misunderstandings.

His efforts showed a commitment to a basic philosophy which he treated like a discovery. He did not present his approach as an absolute knowledge and as perfect. His questions about the nature of human relationships, the nature of empathy, were always directed to the not-yet-known; as if he could see more clearly what he himself had initiated in the light of new experiences. This interest in his own approach was the consequence of a radical vision. It was not the question of the effectiveness of his therapeutic approach which was really in the foreground, but the innovative power of a revolutionary approach which he had formed in his vision of the new human being (Rogers, 1980).

The freedom which he conceded to all others out of his anti-dogmatic attitude meant for him to follow his vision, to commit himself to this vision. And he did this with the same consistency as he presented his anti-dogmatic attitude.

This other side of Rogers comes through in the discipline with which he demonstrated his therapeutic skills. Those who have ever watched Rogers at work, or watched video films of demonstration interviews, have seen that he expressed his therapeutic qualities not only with high skill but also with high discipline. He has thus left an excellent and unmistakable model which is unique in its power of persuasion.

Rogers' commitment is also expressed in his efforts as a theorist. He tried over and over to formulate his theoretical positions ever more clearly and to define his position *vis-à-vis* others (Skinner, Kohut, Erickson or May).

Rogers' commitment is also shown in his despairing patience, to protect his concept of empathy against misunderstandings. It was this empathy which seemed to have shown Rogers that his anti-dogmatic attitude and the generosity arising from it can also be a burden. He was not happy with the term 'reflection of feelings' and reacted in an allergic way every time he heard it (Rogers, 1986). He expected damage to the person-centred approach, 'done by uncritical and unquestioning "disciples"' (Rogers, 1961, p. 15) who used person-centred concepts in right and wrong ways in their

277

missionary enthusiasm to convert others, commenting: 'I have found it difficult to know, at times, whether I have been hurt more by my "friends" or my enemies' (Rogers, 1961, p. 15).

Both motives however – the commitment to the basic approach and philosophy of human relationships and the anti-dogmatic attitude – were crucial for the dissemination of the person-centred approach. The fact that both motives are in a specific tension relationship between freedom and commitment has, however, led to a proneness to crises, because the ambivalences were taken up in an unbalanced and unreflective way.

### UNREFLECTIVE ANTI-DOGMATISM

The anti-dogmatic attitude is sometimes cultivated in an unreflective way. In the name of freedom the person-centred approach is shortened to an unrecognizable communication technique. Under the title 'authenticity and spontaneity' grotesque interaction forms are created, which resemble behavioural disorders rather than a reflected expression of a person-centred attitude. Attempts to find a personal style have sometimes led to a lot of stylistic blunder, to the attempt to sell bad habits as an expression of highest therapeutic competence.

The necessity to relate new concepts and interpretations of person-centred therapy to basic concepts or traditional concepts is sometimes not seen. References to personal experiences (which are not reported in detail) are sometimes the only arguments in theoretical discourses.

### AUTHORITY PROBLEM

I think we have to face the fact that some who follow the person-centred concept have a very unbalanced relationship to authority, including the authority which results from Rogers' approach. This is understandable because the call for independence and for scepticism *vis-à-vis* authorities is backed by an impressive and convincing model in Rogers' own work, an example which is hard to reach but also hard to ignore. The solutions are sometimes found in between imitation and stubborn idiosyncrasy, while boasting the right to develop one's own idea of 'person-centred', even if one cannot present reasonable connections to Rogers' concepts.

## THE DILEMMA WITHIN THE PROFESSIONAL WORLD

The second set of obstacles to the establishment of a clear sense of identity as a person-centred therapist exists in the social and economic conditions in which therapists currently carry out their professional role. Here the competition between different schools reinforces a trend toward instrumentalism and technology. The pressure to be successful directs all therapists towards closed and narrow views of effectiveness which are difficult to square with person-centred principles.

### QUANTITY

One problem is the sheer success of person-centred ideas. Unfortunately, however, the popularity of person-centred therapy training programmes today is not so much a product of deep conviction but rather springs from motives of convenience. The same adage might apply to person-centred therapy which was once used about the English language: the English language is so much liked and so widely used as an international business language and conference language because it can so quickly be spoken so poorly.

In a similar way one suspects that client-centred therapy is often taught primarily, and wrongly, because it is believed to be easy to learn. In fact the idea seems to be that everyone can learn it: it just takes some friendly and understanding person. There are probably in no other therapy form so many who think so soon that they have already mastered it, even without training.

## ESTIMATION BY OTHERS

The crisis also results from the estimation of person-centred therapy by other therapeutic schools. The basic principles of person-centred therapy present a provoking counterpoint to them. Research has shown for instance that the person-centred principles also prove to be valid in other schools. Strangely enough this fact has been used as an argument for the limitation of the person-centred view, the argument being that other therapeutic approaches were always based on person-centred principles anyway. This again represents a shallow misinterpretation of the approach.

The disappearing convincing force of person-centred therapy, therefore, appears in the view that person-centred therapy is a pale approach for everything, does not have any in-depth effects, and is only useful for minor crises of life; it is something for beginners, higher qualifications can only be found in other therapeutic approaches.

These misunderstandings reflect very serious identity problems, which have a number of side-effects: a disappearing convincing force to the outside, deprecation by other therapy schools, and – probably even worse – a disappearing discernment within followers of the approach which reduces person-centred therapy to a drill-ground of mechanical forms of intervention. Hence the relevance of the debate on what it actually does mean to be person-centred (Cain, 1986).

## THE PSYCHO-BOOM AND THE PSYCHO-MARKET

In recent years there has been an upsurge of interest in psychology and therapy, a 'psycho-boom' which has created a 'psycho-market'. The dynamics of this psycho-market have also had an impact on the development and the practice of the person-centred approach.

Economic demands and competition between distinct therapeutic schools further reinforce a trend towards instrumentalism and technology. The pressure to be successful directs person-centred therapists towards closed and narrow views of effectiveness.

To sell an approach it has to be packaged in marketable chunks. Novelty sells. The latest technology seems to be just right on the psycho-market. A certain obsession with new psycho-technologies is in. There are hardly any therapists who think that they can manage their work with their first-choice therapy form. New techniques must constantly be found, best of all dramatic ones, since they seem to provide the guarantee for effectiveness. They have various names, but what is common to them all is their mental attitude, which praises the power of technique. Instrumentalism promotes manipulation and is not consistent with the person-centred approach (Farson, 1978; Rowan, 1987).

Related to this same trend is a drift into the kind of linear thinking which suggests that effectiveness of a method is proportional to dosage, that more is better: more congruity, more openness, more closeness, more empathy (Farson, 1978).


## DISCUSSION

So we see that the ambivalence between freedom and commitment inside the person-centred approach, which I tried to describe earlier, which leads to a proneness to crises, is further aggravated by this economic and professional context. The pressure for accommodation with instrumentalism aggravates the identity problems of the person-centred therapist; and the solution is searched for in a therapeutic eclecticism, an eclecticism which seems to offer the possibility of security, recognition and belonging.

Both factors – the confusing ambivalence between anti-dogmatism and commitment and the adaptation to technology and instrumentalistic approaches – create problems in the development of a distinct person-centred identity. The therapist who lacks a strong professional self, who is not grounded in person-centred theory and philosophy and not supported by practical success and professional satisfaction in therapeutic work with clients, is not

281

able to protect his professional identity against these influencing forces.

Beginners especially are exposed to these problems. In the case of therapeutic failures or helplessness in therapeutic situations, they become vulnerable to quick introjections of direct or underhanded devaluations of the person-centred approach by others, and succumb to the temptation to adopt manipulative or directive techniques incompatible with person-centred values. They suffer from their lack of brilliance even if they do a good job, because the person-centred approach does not offer them controlling techniques that demonstrate their psychological power as therapists, nor an extensive theory with which to dazzle others.

These processes create tensions in the professional identity of person-centred therapists, which can be reduced by leaving the basic principles of person-centred therapy and by adopting techniques from other schools, which promise to equip the therapist with more power and more visible influence on the client than original person-centred therapy does.

Let us take a short, but more detailed look at the inner processes which support these identity problems. The person-centred approach, or person-centred training programmes, tend to attract people who have problems of self-confidence, who are therefore very little protected against deprecation. The pressure of adjustment and competition on the psycho-market does not challenge but rather increases this lack of orientation in a negative way. The person (colleague) who is deprecating gains power by doing this and paradoxically gains esteem and is taken seriously. The unprotected beginner takes the deprecation as competent judgement. And the introjection of this negative evaluation by the other quickly leads to the adoption of a more eclectic stance.

The result lies in the trend of the psycho-market and supports it. A further vulnerability comes from the experience of trainees that the person-centred approach does not have very much to offer to make the function of the therapist brilliant and imposing. It does not have significant techniques to show that the therapist has the power, gives strong impulses and clearly controls the process. There is also no magic theoretic vocabulary which can be used to cover up failures.

The only thing with which a person-centred therapist can impress others in a successful therapy is his or her client. The progress of the client is impressive, next to which the efforts of the therapist seem very little. In a good therapy the dynamics which are shown by the client block the view to the therapist – in particular to outsiders. This phenomenon is shown in comments on therapy sessions in which a client becomes more and more open and differentiated. The uniformed are likely to say, 'That's really easy with this client, he is like an open book.' The possibility that the same client would develop opposition and defence mechanisms with a directive and less sensitive therapist taking the process in a completely different direction is not taken into account and so the competence of the person-centred therapist who makes it look so easy is underrated.

To summarize: I have discussed some components of the professional identity problem of person-centred therapists:

1. Unbalanced solutions of the ambivalence between anti-dogmatism and freedom on the one hand and commitment to person-centred basic principles on the other lead to theoretical and practical disorientation.
2. The dynamics of the psycho-market and the economic context of the therapy profession support a trend towards instrumentalism and technology, structure and leadership, which put a pressure to adapt upon person-centred therapists.
3. Problems of self-confidence of trainees and also some experienced therapists concerning their own approach make them vulnerable and open to conditions of worth incompatible with person-centred values.
4. Finally, because person-centred therapy needs respectful, sensitive and non-intrusive therapists, who proceed at the client's pace and trust the client's resources, it does not offer impressive techniques, which flatter the therapist and make his or her influence on the client visible. Practitioners tend to suffer from this

lack of brilliance which opens a new domain of vulnerability.

The interaction of these components creates a proneness to identity problems in person-centred therapists which supports a tendency to eclectic instrumentalism.

These are my ideas on some problems of developing a person-centred identity in trainees and professional therapists. Let me finish with a paradox. I think we must accept that no school of therapy will ever reach the whole truth. But I think it is also true, as Rogers said back in 1951: 'Truth is not arrived at by concessions from differing schools of thought' (Rogers, 1951, p. 8).

## REFERENCES

CAIN, D. (1986), 'What does it mean to be "person-centred"?' *Person-Centered Review*, 1, 3, 251–56.

FARSON, R. (1978), 'The technology of humanism', *Journal of Humanistic Psychology*, 18, 2, 5–35.

ROGERS, C. R. (1951), *Client-Centered Therapy: its current practice, implications, and theory.* Boston: Houghton Mifflin.

ROGERS, C. R. (1957), 'The necessary and sufficient conditions of therapeutic personality change', *Journal of Consulting Psychology* 21, 95–103.

ROGERS, C. R. (1961), *On Becoming a Person.* Boston: Houghton Mifflin.

ROGERS, C. R. (1980), *A Way of Being.* Boston: Houghton Mifflin.

ROGERS, C. R. (1986), 'Reflecting of feelings', *Person-Centered Review*, 1, 4, 375–77.

ROGERS, C. R. (1987), 'Comments on the issue of equality in psychotherapy', *Journal of Humanistic Psychology*, 27, 1, 38–40.

ROWAN, J. (1987), 'Nine humanistic heresies', *Journal of Humanistic Psychology*, 27, 2, 141–47.

# Notes on Contributors

**Svend Andersen**, Psychological Laboratory, Copenhagen University, Denmark.

**Caroline Beech** is a director of the Eigenwelt Centre for Phenomenological Psychotherapy in Newcastle-upon-Tyne. She is interested in the integration of therapy and the arts. She is currently also engaged in research with women with eating disorders.

**Jerold Bozarth** is professor and director of the Person-Centered Studies Project at the University of Georgia in the USA. He is co-editor of the international *Person-Centered Journal* and has published a very large number of contributions to the theory of the person-centred approach and the field of counselling and mental health.

**David Brazier** is a writer and therapist resident in the north of England. He is a director of the Eigenwelt Centre for Phenomenological Psychotherapy and its associated French project, the Amida Centre. He is author of *A Guide to Psychodrama* and a number of papers on phenomenological and east—west approaches to psychotherapy.

**Ann Weiser Cornell** is a teacher of focusing and editor of the newsletter *The Focusing Connection*.

**Ned Gaylin** is a professor at the University of Maryland and director there of the graduate programme in marriage and family therapy. He is married with four children. He has been a pioneer of person-centred approaches to family therapy and also has a particular interest in the study and enhancement of creativity.

**Len Holdstock** is a clinical psychologist at the Free University in Amsterdam. Born in South Africa, he later became a student of Carl Rogers at the University of Wisconsin, then worked with Rogers as a Visiting Fellow of the Center for Studies of the Person in La Jolla, California, subsequently arranging Rogers' first visit to Africa in 1982. His publications include contributions on research into brain functioning and REM sleep, on indigenous African healing methods, education and transpersonal art.

**Robert Hutterer** works at the University of Vienna, Austria. His interests are humanistic psychology, the philosophy of science and psychotherapy. He was a co-founder of a training programme for person-centred therapy and counselling in Vienna and he is currently involved in organizing a major international conference on client-centred and experiential psychotherapy.

**Mia Leijssen** works as a therapist at the Centre for Client-Centred Therapy at the Catholic University of Leuven in Belgium where she has a practice in individual and group psychotherapy. She also works as a teacher of focusing.

**Germain Lietaer** is Professor in Clinical Psychology at the Catholic University of Leuven, Belgium. He teaches group psychotherapy, client-centred therapy and process research in psychotherapy and is director of the counselling centre where he is part of a team offering a postgraduate training in client-centred therapy.

**Joao Marques-Teixeira** is a psychiatrist and psychotherapist and holds a professorship at the University of Oporto in Portugal where he has been developing a client-centred psychodrama option as well as helping to found a Portuguese association for the person-centred approach. He has published a number of research articles.

**Charles Merrill**, Department of Psychology, Sonoma State University, California.

**Ebrahim Saley** was born in South Africa which he left in 1976, going to study in Cairo and then in Amsterdam. During his stay in The Netherlands he has been active in promoting inter-racial dialogue within the South African expatriate community. He is vice president of the South African Community and Cultural Centre in the Netherlands.

**Ruth Sanford** was Carl Rogers' colleague and close companion in the later years of his life and travelled with him on his important ventures to South Africa and Russia. Together they advanced the application of Rogers' ideas, developing work aimed at resolving cross-cultural conflicts through the human encounter. She continues to be a leading voice for person-centred principles and their further growth.

**Greet Vanaerschot** is a therapist at the counselling centre of the Catholic University of Leuven in Belgium.